For any leader in need of a solution to the burnout crisis in their organization, *The Busy Brain Cure* provides a scientific solution that cost-effective and easy to implement for individuals and teams. Romie serves as our Chief Wellness Officer, and her unique pertise in neurology, integrative medicine, and mindfulness have lped to create a cultural movement within the organization."

—Will Loughran, president of Evolution Hospitali

e *Busy Brain Cure* is the solution to the toxic hustle culture in the kplace that is fueling anxiety, difficulty focusing, and FOMO ut work. Bringing together brain science and powerful client sformation stories, Dr. Romie shares an 8-week plan to heal out that founders and leaders need to address focus and uctivity."

—Suneera Madhani, founder of Stax and CEO Scho

is a program that dismantles the toxic diet culture and honors l diversity of foods while using a protocol to reduce stress eating. sy *Brain Cure* uses researched microhabits known as brainSHIFT simple and easy to implement for busy professionals and to help improve your ability to focus and daytime energy."

—Kanchan Koya, PhD, Harvard-trained doctor in biomedicin
and Chief Spice Mama and founder of Radical Vitali

workplace culture starts and ends with team members feeling and supported. One of the best investments an organization is in tools and resources that help associates manage stress, r work-life balance, and prioritize mental well-being. By ting practices from *The Busy Brain Cure* into our corporate wellness initiatives, we've been able to equip and empower with science-based programs that heal the root cause of d help boost engagement."

—Ann Christenson, chief human resource offic
of Aimbridge Hospitali

Praise for *The Busy Brain Cure*

"*The Busy Brain Cure* will transform how individuals and
organizations approach the outdated conversation on die
stress, and burnout. Dr. Romie combines her authority as
neurologist, holistic health expert, and corporate Chief V
Officer to lead a researched, comprehensive, easy-to-i
program called brainSHIFT. brainSHIFT will help you to
sugar cravings, curb stress eating, and tame anxiety s
focus, feel energized, and sleep through the night."

—**JJ Virgin, CNS, CHFI, Nutrition & Fi**
***New York Times* best**

"For any leader searching for a solution to the workplac
and burnout crisis, *The Busy Brain Cure* offers a compel
based program based on the latest brain science. Dr. F
authority as a physician, Chief Wellness Officer, and co
leader has helped countless individuals and teams ref
relationship to stress and build wellness cultures."

—**John Murphy, CEO, C**

"*The Busy Brain Cure* isn't just a solution; it's a rev
the CEOs, executives, and entrepreneurs feeling
relentless cycles of stress, anxiety, and burnout:
a transformative path for healing the root caus
expertise in neurology and integrative medicir
wisdom, and captivating storytelling to guide
balanced, sustainable way of working, leadir

—**Natalie MacNeil, Emmy Award—winni**
author of *The Rituals*, and foun

"If you identify as creatively fulfilled but
that won't stop, *The Busy Brain Cure* del
have been searching for. In true Dr. Ror
won't be told to meditate for an hour a
aspirations, rather you will get a medi
literally reduces inflammation in your
better, sharpen your focus and do th

—**Pamela Slim, award-w**

THE
BUSY
BRAIN
CURE

THE EIGHT-WEEK PLAN TO FIND FOCUS, TAME ANXIETY, AND SLEEP AGAIN

DR. ROMIE MUSHTAQ, MD

HANOVER
SQUARE
PRESS

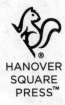

HANOVER
SQUARE
PRESS™

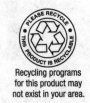

Recycling programs
for this product may
not exist in your area.

ISBN-13: 978-1-335-00711-7

The Busy Brain Cure

Hanover Square Press
22 Adelaide St. West, 41st Floor
Toronto, Ontario M5H 4E3, Canada
HanoverSqPress.com
BookClubbish.com

Printed in U.S.A.

Dedicated to all of my teachers—
from my proud years in the American public school education system
to the professors in my medical training
and the teachings of the global healing community
and especially for the wisdom and patience of all my aunties.

TABLE OF CONTENTS

Introduction 9

SECTION ONE—Busy Brain: Stuck in the Stress-Success Cycle **21**

Are You Stuck on the Stress-Success Cycle? 23

brainDUMP Chapter 1 Summary 38

Signs That Your Stress Created a Busy Brain 40

brainDUMP Chapter 2 Summary 54

Busy Brain Cure—One Size Does Not Fit All 56

brainDUMP Chapter 3 Summary 67

How Do You Cure a Busy Brain? 70

brainDUMP Chapter 4 Summary 87

SECTION TWO—The Scientific Cause of Your Busy Brain and the brainSHIFT Acronym. **91**

S: Sleep and the Circadian Rhythm of a Busy Brain 93

brainDUMP Chapter 5 Summary 110

H: Hormones in a Busy Brain 112

brainDUMP Chapter 6 Summary 132

I: Inflammation, Sugar and Caffeine in a Busy Brain 134

brainDUMP Chapter 7 Summary 150

F: Food and Fat as brainFUEL for a Busy Brain 152

brainDUMP Chapter 8 Summary 167

T: Technology and a Busy Brain 168

brainDUMP Chapter 9 Summary 186

SECTION THREE—The 8-Week brainSHIFT Protocol 189

brainSHIFT Protocol, Week 1—Starting Goals Instead of Self-Judgments 191

brainWORK Week 1 202

brainSHIFT Protocol, Week 2—7-Day Sleep Challenge. . . 204

brainWORK Week 2 214

brainSHIFT Protocol, Week 3—Digital Detox 222

brainWORK Week 3 231

brainSHIFT Protocol, Week 4—brainPAUSE 233

brainWORK Week 4 243

brainSHIFT Protocol, Week 5—Biohack Your Nutrition. . 246

brainWORK Week 5 253

brainSHIFT Protocol, Week 6—Fuel, Energy and Focus . . 257

brainWORK Week 6 263

brainSHIFT Protocol, Week 7—Superbrain Superhormones. . 266

brainWORK Week 7 276

brainSHIFT Protocol, Week 8—Putting It All Together . . 280

brainWORK Week 8 285

Appendix A **293**

Appendix B **297**

Appendix C **303**

Bibliography **327**

Acknowledgments **369**

INTRODUCTION

I wrote this book for you, my fellow unapologetic, type A, success-driven professionals. You may have been told to slow down, but the problem is we don't want to slow down. Quite frankly, we do not have the luxury to pause, take a break, or go on a self-care sabbatical. You are the leaders, change-makers, caregivers, single parents, night-school-attending, mortgage-paying adults who live in the real world. A 4-hour workweek? Impossible! The successful people with passion for their purpose whom I've served aren't working 4 hours a week. They are teachers, lawyers, journalists, nurses, techies, finance executives, hotel general managers, airline pilots, accountants, doctors, start-up founders, architects, nonprofit directors, national sales leaders, C-suite executives, bankers, or pharmaceutical representatives, and they have deep, meaningful goals. In consulting with these dedicated, hardworking, and amazing people, I discovered that we all had one thing in common: if one more person told us to "chill" or "go with the flow," we would run over them with our wearable tech and designer shoes.

But inside that purpose-driven life, we also understand that there must be a different way to succeed that doesn't lead to burning ourselves out. After countless years of research as well as my personal experience with burnout and the health issues that stem from it, I became committed to finding a path to success without wearing stress as a badge of honor. We don't have to apologize for our drive, but there are key actions we can take to avoid being overcome by stress and burnout. The answers came in the conversations with many of you in convention hall corridors when I was giving my keynote lectures on stress management. I'm so thankful for all of you who stood in line to talk with me, sometimes for over 2 hours, to tell me about your symptoms and frustrations with the current medical system. I can't tell you the number of people who asked for the cure to their Busy Brain, a term you will come to know intimately through the reading of this book. A Busy Brain is the term I coined for a pattern of neuroinflammation in the brain caused by chronic stress and burnout. Symptoms of a Busy Brain include an inability to focus, anxiety, and difficulty falling and staying asleep.

If up to now you don't know my work and haven't seen one of my keynotes, you might be asking, how do I know if this applies to me? Let's have some Dr. Romie Real Talk. You might have a Busy Brain if any one of these statements resonates with you:

• You can't connect to your personality without a venti dairy-free latte in the morning. If, by chance, the barista used whole milk, then you are Bitter with a capital *B* for the rest of the day.

- You tell me you just drink coffee, but you really chugged three energy drinks, and if I caught you from the stage, you tried to hide the can under your seat. Busted.

- Your day/schedule/task list has been hijacked by a mysterious external force.

- There are too many browser windows open on your computer and in your brain.

- You try to focus on one important task, but the dinging of notifications from your email inbox, messenger channels, and text messages distracts you. It takes 47 minutes to finish a task that should take less than 3 minutes.

- You finally make it to the end of the day and need a glass of wine or three, followed by bourbon to take the edge off.

- If you don't drink alcohol, you are trying the latest fad supplement that some Instagram influencer shared.

- You are wired and tired—you're sure you will sleep well tonight, but when you put your head down on your pillow, you can't shut down the racing thoughts.

- Once again, the ping of a notification pulls your finger to the screen of your phone, and you lose another 92 minutes down the Google research rabbit hole, wondering why you have been researching high-grade plungers for your bathroom.

- When you finally fall asleep, you wake up at 2:37 a.m. or thereabouts and are wide awake. Heck, you may as well knock out some emails or get a load of laundry done before the kids get up.

Be honest. Did you say yes to any of the above?

No judgment from me. As you'll see in this book, I used to suffer from these symptoms but continued to churn and burn. That is, churn through the day and burn the midnight oil. I wore stress as a badge of honor, which led me straight down the path of burnout and eventually required lifesaving surgery. I thought that the system was stacked against me, just like you think the system is stacked against you.

When my brain got lost in my dark hole, the last thing I wanted to hear was, "Everything is going to be fine; just focus on rainbows, butterflies, and puppies." I didn't need another meditation class or to be shamed into another lesson on resilience. Toxic positivity deepened the wounds, and I kept searching for a new way of being that I didn't have access to with the adult survival skills I had then.

Have you been stuck on a stress-success cycle too? Where is the adulting manual to help us pivot, rebuild, and reinvigorate? Heck, right now, you may be scrolling and trolling Instagram for a pseudo-inspirational reel in millennial pink to help your brain cope for the next 47 minutes of that virtual conference call—video off—but hey, can someone help turn your brain back on?

If I could share one message to help jump-start your healing process, my heart wants you to know this:

Your brain is not broken.

Your mind is not a mess.

And hope did not permanently depart your soul.

Busy Brain in a Busy World

Between our schedules, screens, and screaming individuals on the street, our senses are overloaded. There are too many browser windows open on our multiple screens, and in our brains. We no longer live in a world where stressors are temporary and our brains have a chance to reset back to a calm channel.

Instead, stress is chronic, and we can feel helpless as we sink further into burnout. I am here to tell you that living with chronic stress takes its toll on your memory, ability to think, mood, and all aspects of your physical health. Chronic and unchecked stress will cause chronic disease, and it will kill you. It almost killed me, and I'm a brain doctor. I should have known better.

What if I told you that traditional medicine got it wrong? That attention deficit disorder (ADD), anxiety, and insomnia in adults are not three different problems but are all part of one syndrome? I call this syndrome a Busy Brain.

And the problem? Here in the West, we use stimulants like caffeine to energize and focus all day and sedatives like alcohol at night to cope. And when the coffee-wine combination fails, some physicians hand out prescription Adderall to get you through your day and then a sleeping or antianxiety pill at night to help you chill out. We are stuck on a stimulant-sedative cycle, all in the name of success.

And let me be clear right here in the introduction. The cure to a Busy Brain is not a cleanse, a diet, or the next nutrition fad. In fact, when we cure our Busy Brains, we stop stress eating and instead mindfully enjoy comfort food. Yes, this brain doctor is telling you to eat comfort food, and in section two, you will learn why it is the path to not only curing your Busy Brain, but also honoring the diverse people on your teams in the workplace. And go ahead, take a quick peek at the appendix. I'll wait. You'll see we share a sample of the comfort foods from my circle of loved ones for you.

Here's another thing. You don't need another time management technique or productivity tool either. How many self-development books have you read, listened to while working out, or sworn that you would follow, only to feel like it is another to-do list item adding to your stress levels?

brainSHIFT: The Busy Brain Cure

If we don't get the state of our brains straight, we cannot build our dreams or our teams. If we don't start by optimizing our brain function, we'll never be able to optimize our passion, purpose, relationships, and callings. So, yes, this brain doctor is telling you not to apologize for your drive or maybe not even for your 60-hour workweek. It is possible as long as your brain is functioning at capacity, and right now, I haven't met many brains that are (including my own, at times). When we cure our Busy Brains, we can focus, remain calm, sleep, and optimize our performance. How would it feel to be back in control of not only your schedule, but your ability to pay attention, to sleep, to not feel so anxious all the time?

As an award-winning speaker, founder of the brainSHIFT Institute, and Chief Wellness Officer, I've been conducting research with individuals and teams in corporate America specifically on curing their Busy Brains for the past 3 years. For this book, I brought my 20 years of experience as a researcher, doctor of neurology and integrative medicine (add a dash of tech, sass, and soul). We cannot forget to mention the wisdom of my Aunties—they must not be ignored, and how can you with the flashy 22-K yellow-gold necklaces and bracelets they are wearing for this special occasion? My Aunties are elders who were friends with my immigrant parents, and they hailed from different religious and cultural backgrounds. The one thing they had in common was traditional family values, and the openhearted desire to make sure I grew up to become a doctor, and marry well. (Not necessarily in that order.)

And in this book, you will also hear the stories of individuals, teams, and organizations who participated in my brainSHIFT Protocol and were committed to curing their Busy Brains. I also candidly share my journey from Busy Brain to burnout and back again with the help of both Western doctors and global healers.

My cure for the Busy Brain is called the brainSHIFT Protocol. It was developed as I thought back to all the individual patients I had treated in neurology and integrative medicine with similar symptoms. As I successfully treated these patients, I wondered: How can I scale this concept to share it with teams and the public at large? Since 2020, when the global pandemic hit, I was prompted to get creative using technology, so the brainSHIFT 8-week wellness program went online. Not only did we help to restore sleep and a sense of sanity in a time that was, frankly, quite stressful, the teams who participated felt a rejuvenated sense of connection even if they could not be in the office together.

The Busy Brain Cure is not just meant for professionals working from home. A Busy Brain does not have cultural or country-specific boundaries. According to the World Health Organization, 3.6% (about 264 million) of people worldwide have an anxiety disorder. Additionally, 4.6% of females and 2.6% of males globally are affected by anxiety. The *State of the Global Workplace 2022 Report* was conducted in 116 countries by Gallup and indicated that 43% of employees experience workplace stress.

In over 120 virtual global presentations that I gave between 2020 and 2022, no one wanted this brain doctor to tell them to "eat berries and breathe, and everything will be just fine." I needed to help find a solution for individuals and a strategy for corporate teams.

So what is brainSHIFT? I define a brainSHIFT as a series of microhabits to implement that have the biggest impacts on your brain and physical health. The "SHIFT" in brainSHIFT is an acronym for the five key areas that are responsible for the root cause of a Busy Brain in most individuals.

S = sleep
H = hormones
I = markers of inflammation
F = food as fuel
T = technology

Every Busy Brain is unique, and together we will figure out the key area for you to focus on between sleep, hormones, inflammation, food, and technology. You may not need to cover each area, but starting with a solid sleep foundation (chapter 5) is essential on the path to taming your Busy Brain.

How to Use This Book, the brainSHIFT Protocol, and Tame Your Busy Brain

You didn't get here overnight, so I will not lie and tell you there is a fancy brain scan or overpriced supplement to offer you a quick fix. There is no on-off switch on your brain that you can access by meditation or buying an overpriced pair of house slippers. What I am going to offer you is years of field testing, the latest medical research, stories, and the cure for a Busy Brain to help you move forward. In this book, you are offered the 8-week plan to help you find focus, tame your anxiety, and sleep again. I include bonuses such as self-assessment questionnaires, labs to discuss with your doctor, and the brainSHIFT Protocol to start weekly microhabits to tame your Busy Brain.

In section one, we will take a journey to understand the stress-success cycle, how chronic stress can lead to neuro-inflammation, disease, and specifically to a Busy Brain.

In section two, we break down the scientific research into the root causes of a Busy Brain, ranging from a disruption in your circadian rhythm, to your hormones, to the role of technology.

And in section three, we will walk you through the researched and tested 8-week brainSHIFT Protocol to cure your Busy Brain.

Through this book, I want to offer you both hope and solutions. We no longer have to live with low-key anxiety, chug caffeine all day to focus, drink half a bottle of red wine at night to calm down, or allow our endless to-do lists to rob us of our sanity.

Back in 2010, as I started the search for a cure for a Busy Brain, *burnout* wasn't a widely recognized term. People like me were written off as "too weak to handle the pressure." Today an estimated 82% of the American workforce has symptoms of burnout—but neither you nor I are just another sad statistic. We are the experts, innovators, and leaders of our families, communities, and organizations. Somewhere on the path from a Busy Brain to burnout, there is an opportunity to pause, self-reflect, and take measured action.

If you had told me as I lay in the dark place my life had become due to burnout, that one day my brain would be functioning better than when I was in medical school, I wouldn't have believed you. In fact, I could not have imagined this type of peak performance. I started as a sleep-deprived and frazzled doctor. I cured my Busy Brain and brainSHIFTed to become an entrepreneur who woke up energized and in control of my inbox, calendar, and emotions. I now have laser-sharp focus to live my driven, passion-filled life as an award-winning speaker, female founder, and Chief Wellness Officer scaling mindfulness and wellness programs to over 7,000 employees.

So if you feel like you lost control or ended up burned out, I want you to know:

Your brain is not broken.

Your mind is not a mess.

Hope did not depart your soul.

It's an honor to be your guide on the path forward. Now, let's turn the page together, and brainSHIFT.

Dr. Romie

SECTION ONE

Busy Brain: Stuck on the
Stress-Success Cycle

1

Are You Stuck on the Stress-Success Cycle?

Girl, Maybelline, you lied to me. This mascara ain't waterproof.

I sobbed as I navigated Interstate 94, and when I glanced into the rearview mirror, my appearance just made me cry harder as black rivers of said mascara ran down my cheeks. The heated seat of my smoky mica granite Lexus IS 350 was not providing its usual comfort. I took a deep breath and glided over the three icy highway lanes toward the exit for the hospital where I was an attending physician and professor of neurology. I didn't even know why I was crying; I was just so damned tired. I'd worked my entire life to become a doctor and dreamed of creating a better life for female epilepsy patients.

"I love my job. I love my job. I love my job," I whispered into my rearview mirror.

Don't I?

My Italian silk black suit and overpriced Jimmy Choo stilettos could no longer hide the fact that I was not as pulled together as the designer labels would suggest. It was 6:42 a.m., and already the beeper was buzzing for another stat consult in the neuro-critical-care ICU. I reached for my breakfast, but the only thing I could find was a stale, half-frozen piece of KitKat sitting in the console. I ate it anyway.

How in the hell did I get here?

I had followed (almost) every rule given to me since I wore my plastic neon-red-and-yellow Fisher Price stethoscope on my first day of preschool. I'd grown up with one success mantra from my immigrant father, who had whispered it to me in the newborn nursery and every day after that during my childhood: "We have one daughter, and you will become a doctor."

Any other life-guiding principles from my circle of elders led back to that one goal.

"Go study your math and science. Otherwise, how will you get into medical school?"

"Hooo-hai-hai, future doctors do NOT say those curse words."

"We pray that one day you will find a suitable husband. After all, you went to medical school."

Like any other working adult in the United States, my days were balanced between checking off items on my to-do list and acquiring labels, achievements, and more shoes. To the outside world, I had every title expected of me—doctor, professor, researcher, and dutiful daughter. I married well and then promptly divorced 3 years later with even more flair. And just when one might start to doubt my pristine facade, my overpriced designer high heels would click-clack down the hospital corridors and snap any doubters back to attention. I was a bona fide STEMinist in Stilettos who had arrived to take control of the situation.

While on the outside I kept up the facade of self-control, internally, it felt like my brain cells were on fire. No matter how much caffeine I drank, I couldn't seem to focus or have enough energy to get through the day. If any emotion dared to destroy my doctor-in-control image, I would immediately self-medicate with more chocolate. I was wired and tired and consistently robbed of a routine sleep schedule. When I put my head down on my pillow, seventy-two warring conversations took over as I tried to process my day, judge my actions, and add to my never-ending to-do list. What was controlling the on-off switch in my brain to stop the insanity and restore order?

Nothing, I suppose.

I was a faithful follower of the churn and burn daily spiritual practice—the norm for any of us employed in academic medicine. Churn all cylinders during the day, and burn the midnight oil. Stress ourselves out until we reach another level of success, then rinse and repeat. I was definitely stuck on the stress-success cycle.

I pulled my Lexus into the hospital parking lot, chocolate from the KitKat still on my fingers, and mustered up the courage to get out of my car and strategically keep my balance on the icy sidewalk leading to the sliding doors of the neuroscience division.

That's the moment I started to have searing chest pain.

What I know 16 years later, beyond a shadow of a doubt, is that we can no longer wear stress as a badge of honor, which was what I was doing as I walked into work every day. All those years ago when I drove my Lexus on that icy freeway, we didn't have terms like *burnout, chronic stress*, or *employee well-being*. After all this time, I've learned that chronic stress is toxic and destroys the structure and function of our brains and bodies. We can no longer sacrifice our health to achieve our goals in the pursuit of success. Chronic stress over time actually WILL kill you. Is that too bold a statement? I am not being a drama queen. It almost killed me.

brainSCIENCE Break
Are You Stuck on a Stress-Success Cycle?

Have you ever asked yourself, "Why can't I be truly calm or happy in my life? What's missing?" Only to have your inner voice immediately answer, "Maybe if I meet my quota for my sales goal this quarter, then I'll be happy." Or, "Maybe when I finish that next big remodeling project in the house, I'll finally be able to calm down."

Like the success-driven professional you have become, you've set your SMART goals, used the GTD method, and put myriad other structures and systems in place to manage yourself and your output. You also stress, obsess, and worry until you achieve whatever goal you're working toward in the moment. But invariably, that nagging feeling comes right back—something is missing. You're not feeling calm anymore or focused. You ask yourself what else is on your to-do list. You'll focus on that because it will make you feel better. But it doesn't.

That, my dear reader, is being stuck on a stress-success

cycle. And listen, as a triple board-certified physician and C-suite-level executive, I am not here to tell you that striving for success is wrong. But what if I told you we could strive for success in our personal and professional lives without stressing ourselves out?

I'm here to tell you that you *are* stuck on the success-stress cycle if you subscribe to the "success at any cost" mantra while wearing your stress as a badge of honor. You have trained your brain to believe that if you could just check off one more item on your never-ending to-do list then you will have achieved inner peace. What's so wrong with that? Well, instead of the inner peace that you're so sure is at the end of all those completed check marks (a pipe dream, at best), you start having back pain, acid reflux, a lost libido, or a panic attack. To boot, you end up ghosting your primary care physician because they claimed that you now have high blood pressure, borderline diabetes mellitus, or an irregular heart rhythm.

Eventually, still stuck on the success-stress cycle, you may even start to develop symptoms of chronic disease in your heart, stomach, lungs, and joints. But, hey, not a thing feels off. Then suddenly, you drop to the ground from a cardiac arrest. Stress can not only derail your plans for success, chronic stress will kill you if you don't address it.

Before you start to panic, I want you to know that it is possible to achieve your goals, be ambitious, and succeed without falling into the pattern of chronic stress, burnout, and ill health. The first step I invite you to take is often the most difficult—it's simply self-awareness. Ultimately, it is your decision, and your decision alone, to get off the stress-success cycle.

What's Stress Got to Do with It Anyway?

When someone starts by simply admitting to me that they are stressed out, it is not uncommon for their defense mechanism to be, "Dr. Romie, who *isn't* stressed in today's modern work world?"

If we were sitting down together one-on-one, I would want to ask you:

1. Have you been stuck on the stress-success cycle for a short period due to a deadline at work?

2. Or are you living with stress all the time due to strains on finances, your relationship, your health, or perhaps something else?

3. Or do you feel like you are always stressed out about life, and then more struggles keep piling on top?

Stress is defined by the World Health Organization as any change that causes physical, emotional, or psychological strain. Any of these types of stress can cause your well-being to deteriorate in one or more of these areas:

- Brain function (cognition)

- Emotional well-being (mental health)

- Function of your body (physical health)

- Sense of self in relation to the world (spiritual health)

When we think about how stress will impact our health,

it is first important to understand that there are not only different types of stress. Stress is also classified by the duration of the stressor. Standard psychology classifies stress into these three types:

1. Acute stress

2. Acute episodic stress

3. Chronic stress

Acute stress results from your body's reaction to a new or challenging situation. This is the feeling you get from an approaching deadline or when you narrowly avoid being hit by a car. In this case, scientists agree a little bit of stress is a normal reaction to make our brains focus, be motivated, or push through procrastination. We can even experience acute stress due to something we enjoy, like riding a roller coaster. Acute stress is classified as short-term. Usually, your stress hormones, emotions, and body will return to a normal state within minutes to hours through the relaxation response in your brain.

The second type of stress is acute episodic stress. Acute episodic stress is when acute stresses (as defined above) happen frequently. You feel like you are constantly moving from one crisis to another. One example of acute episodic stress is having tight work deadlines that happen on a recurring basis without a break. Another example is the frequent high-stress situations experienced by some professionals, such as healthcare workers. Doctors, nurses, and other healthcare workers are repeatedly at the bedside of different patients in a potentially critical state, revving up stress hormones and then repeating the cycle with each patient seen in the emergency room, intensive care unit, or clinic. With acute episodic stress, we don't get time to return to a relaxed and calm state, so the effects of the high-frequency acute stresses accumulate.

Last but not least is chronic stress. Chronic stress results from stressors that continue for an extended period of time and can feel never-ending. Examples include constantly fighting with your life partner, facing insurmountable debt, or living with a chronic disease. In chronic stress, we have difficulty seeing any way to improve or change the situation. In the face of chronic stress, trying temporary relaxation measures like a nap, short meditation, or exercise often doesn't feel like it helps to get us out of stress. Once again, a quick fix or an on-off switch for the brain doesn't exist.

One important item of note in our discussion of stress and its classifications is the idea that "stress is good for you." I want to clear up any confusion here and now around that statement that has been touted in recent years. When you hear that phrase, please understand that they are talking about acute stress, which, as noted above, helps you to push through a deadline, or allows your reflexes to take action quickly. For example, let's say you're driving in winter weather and hit a patch of ice and start skidding. "Stress is good for you" in this situation because the acute stress will allow you to navigate the ice with your brain on high alert and all your reflexes focused. In this book, we're going to target the last two types of stress: acute episodic and chronic stress. Those are the two that I'm worried about, because these types of stress can kill you.

Acute episodic and chronic stress create havoc in our brains and bodies. I want you to think of your brain as having an airport traffic control tower. At a busy airport, the airport traffic control tower oversees the operations of the cabin (in-flight experience), below-plane operations, and above ground (airport) operations. In the same way, our brain has an airport traffic control center that oversees operations in our brain and all of the organ systems in our body.

Your Brain as an Airport Traffic Control Tower

Fourteen years after pushing through the sobbing moments in my car, I found myself in a luxurious affair with my travel boyfriend, Delta Airlines. In 2019, they even gave me the elusive diamond—Diamond Medallion status, that is. I knew we'd taken our relationship to the next level in 2022 when Delta Airlines invited me to meet the family of employees at the mother ship: Hartsfield-Jackson Atlanta International Airport (ATL).

When I woke up on the morning of the big day, the joy and excitement I'd felt over the invitation was clouded in my Busy Brain by the judgmental voices of the Aunties in my head: *"Hai hai, you are a visiting dignitary and guest at their airport. What a big honor Delta Airlines is giving you. You will represent our whole family. Fifty-one years ago, your mother came on a big plane like that from Asia to America when she married your father. What are you going to wear? You come from a good family, so do not bring us shame. You must at a minimum wear proper jewels and something silk."*

As I dressed for my big "date," I heeded the internal guidance (ahem...criticism) of my elders and put on my finest pearls, 22-K gold earrings, and a rose pink silk blouse. When I arrived, I met Rondah Smart, Delta Airlines' ATL Worldport Manager for Employee Engagement and Communications. To her credit she kept her stoic composure as she covered my silk and pearls with a neon-green vest five sizes too big. Plastered across the front of the vest in shiny silver were the words "Delta Visitor." What was more impressive than her stoicism was her compassion and care when she stuck the neon-green earplugs into my ears above my 22-K gold hoops.

Of course, my Busy Brain had conveniently forgotten the critical detail that we would be outside, where the bitter December Atlanta winds would pierce through my fine silk and neon vest as I stood on the tarmac of gate T8. Even with the cold, I stood in awe, saluting the pilots while watching the super tug cart pull the 757 Boeing out of the gate onto the tarmac. To stand underneath the belly of that plane was a life list moment.

Until my "date" with my travel boyfriend that day, I'd had no idea that with one gust of wind, one lightning strike, or one major snow or thunderstorm, this carefully controlled symphony of operations could become chaotic, and a ground stop could be ordered. A ground stop is mandated by the Federal Aviation Authority (FAA) in the airport traffic control tower to ensure no employees are on the tarmac in dangerous weather, nor are any planes attempting to land or take off with poor visibility.

Further, if a ground stop is ordered by the FAA at the ATL traffic control tower, you have just hit the pause button at one of the world's busiest airports. How long do you think it takes for Los Angeles International Airport (LAX) or London Heathrow International Airport (LHR) to be impacted by a ground stop at ATL? Within just a few seconds, the chaos of cancellations and delays spreads to the global airspace, impacting passengers and crews, and causing planes to be delayed or diverted elsewhere.

Our brain and bodies function the same way when we are trying to push operations through. Episodic stress is like a temporary slowdown of one runway at the airport due to the congestion of incoming and outgoing planes taxiing to the right terminal. Piling on acute stress after acute stress for long periods of time causes a chronically stressed brain, which is akin to a complete ground stop. It's not unlike a blizzard coming through ATL. There is now diminishing visibility, it's dangerous for employees to be out on the tarmac, and all below-plane operations slow down or come to a complete halt.

Effect of Stress on Your Brain's and Body's Operations

Your brain also has a fight, flight, or freeze response. Known as the stress response, this is a how your brain responds to any event it perceives as harmful, an attack, or a threat to your survival. This stress response was first described by Dr. Walter Bradford Cannon and is known as the Cannon-Bard theory. The Cannon-Bard theory proposes that your brain's airport traffic control center (the amygdala) processes what you see and hear, translating possible danger to the airport gates (the hypothalamus). In simple terms, the stress response then releases stress hormones that signal you to either freeze, fight, or take flight.

When a winter storm is going to threaten or create harm to the people and operations of ATL airport, the FAA in the airport traffic control tower sends a signal to the other key areas of the airport, known as a ground stop. Until it is safe to resume operations, no planes can take off or land at the airport. Employees who work on the tarmac in below-plane operations also have to go indoors to safety. What appears to a passenger as being stuck in the airport is actually a carefully crafted symphony of operations to keep everyone safe.

When we experience ongoing episodic stress (instead of acute temporary stress), the amygdala acts like the traffic control tower if it were *constantly* sending out a distress signal—the employees at all the airport gates start shifting operations to emergency mode. It is not just the brains of the operation that switch into this crisis mode, but so does the rest of our crew, the body.

Then the hypothalamus activates the autonomic nervous system by sending signals through the sympathetic nerves to the adrenal glands. This is known as our hypothalamic-pituitary-adrenal axis (HPA axis). Our adrenal glands produce key chemicals and hormones that keep our bodies fueled. Under stress, the adrenal glands respond by pumping these chemicals and hormones (cortisol and adrenaline) into the bloodstream. As these hormones circulate through the body, they bring on several physiological changes that signal distress.

1. The heart beats faster than average, pushing blood to the muscles, brain, and other vital organs.

2. The blood pressure also goes up. The person undergoing these changes also starts to breathe more rapidly.

3. Small airways in the lungs open wide. This way, the lungs can take in as much oxygen as possible with each breath.

4. Extra oxygen is sent to the brain, increasing alertness. Sight, hearing, and other senses become sharper.

5. Meanwhile, adrenaline triggers the release of blood sugar (glucose) and fats from temporary storage sites in the body. These nutrients flood into the bloodstream, supplying energy to all our body parts.

It's important to remember that, just like flying through different global airports, every person's body is different, and so is how each individual sees the impact of episodic and chronic stress. Physiological changes can vary from one person to the next, and we each have to understand our own patterns.

When you fly to various airports, they all have different architecture, while key functions operate the same. This is the same with the human brain, our personalities, and ability to cope with stress. What makes your brain's airport traffic control tower panic or shut down can be different than someone else who might have steady-state operations.

Our brain's airport traffic control tower perceives threats differently compared to other people's brains. This is why two people can experience the same situation and may not experience the same stress response, if any at all. For example, two people may hear a toxic coworker yell in the middle of a meeting. One might feel sick to their stomach or may be annoyed by the angry colleague, while the other person doesn't react at all. It doesn't even faze them. As humans, it is normal to have different stress reactions to the same thing; some people perceive a threat, whereas others don't. Another example is public speaking. While 90% of the population fears public speaking, thus inducing a stress response, there are 10%, like myself, who find joy in public speaking—thus it doesn't elicit a strong stress response.

I often joke that my stress relief and relaxation come through research and reading. The habit of reading encyclopedias was instilled in me by my mother and Aunties so they'd be less stressed with me constantly underfoot asking questions. If I had more time, I'd pursue a PhD in psycho-neuro-immuno-endocrinology. Say that five times fast—for most, that repetition is an example of an acute stressor. For me—utter bliss.

It's fascinating to research how emotions and your mood (psycho) change the structure and function of the brain (neuro), thus shifting the body's entire immune system (immuno), and the role of every organ system's hormones (endocrinology). Psycho-neuro-immuno-endocrinology. Stress doesn't just hijack your mood. Through decades of research, we know that emotions change how your brain functions (sleep, memory) and your physical health (digestion, hormones, immune system, muscle tension).

In all three types of stress, the limbic system is the seat of the stress response and where emotions are processed. I want to reiterate that once the amygdala (part of the limbic system) is stimulated by acute, episodic, or chronic stress, it sends a distress signal to the hypothalamus. The HPA axis is then activated. In acute stress, at some point within minutes to hours the relaxation response is elicited—the parasympathetic response to reverse the acute stress effects.

In episodic and chronic stress, there is no chance for the relaxation response to fully bring the brain and body back to homeostasis. The hypothalamus and pituitary glands in the brain are responsible for maintaining the homeostasis of every organ system in the body. There are over fifty different hormones in your brain and body that make sure every organ system is working in harmony. When the HPA axis is activated under stress, glucocorticoids and catecholamines surge. In prolonged stress, the HPA axis continuously stimulates your sympathetic nervous system.

What happens when your sympathetic nervous system is accelerated chronically? With constant stimulation in chronic stress, the sympathetic nervous system will elevate your heart rate and blood pressure, cause muscle tension, inflame your joints, and wreak havoc with your digestion.

I've been there, 16 years ago, as I walked through the sliding doors of the neuroscience division and had that searing chest pain. Little did I know that I was experiencing acute chronic stress in my job as a physician. I was only in my early thirties. Another thing I didn't know back then was that my chest pain was worsening due to the stress my brain's airport traffic control tower could not control…and it was wreaking havoc with my mood, sleep, and digestion. It would be years before I pieced together the puzzle of my symptoms and my personal history to find the solution to maintain homeostasis in the airport traffic control tower of my brain.

brainDUMP Chapter 1 Summary

- You are stuck on a stress-success cycle if you constantly feel stressed trying to achieve your goals, only to start the process all over again on a new goal, task, or to-do list item.

- Depending on the duration and frequency, stress is classified as acute stress, acute episodic stress, or chronic stress.

- Acute episodic stress and chronic stress lead to symptoms that destroy your mental health, cognitive health, physical health, and spiritual well-being.

- Ongoing episodic and chronic stress leads to disease and can kill you.

- Your brain has a system that functions like an airport traffic control tower. This part of your brain controls operations in the rest of your brain and every organ system in your body.

- Under acute episodic and chronic stress, operations in your brain and body can slow down or come to a halt—known as the stress response.

quickSHIFT: Take Fast Action Now

Take a moment now to ask yourself, are you stuck on a stress-success cycle?

Self-Awareness Exercise

1. Do you feel like you have to push yourself at all costs in order to obtain your goals, finish a task, or succeed?

2. Where did this pattern start?

3. What symptoms do you start to feel when stress is pushing you over the edge?

4. Are you ready to take the first step toward breaking this stress-success cycle?

5. Can you think of a time when you succeeded at something important in your life without having to be under a long period of stress?

2

Signs that Your Stress Created a Busy Brain

The chest pain I experienced back in 2007 as I tottered across the ice in my stilettos started right behind the strap in the middle of my La Perla black lace bra—a rapidly ascending fire rising to my throat and searing straight through to the middle of my back. Moments later, a darkness overtook me, and I couldn't breathe. I broke into a sweat. I recovered and went to work, but from that day on these symptoms got more frequent, would haunt me, and would sneak up on me when I least expected it. On a day-to-day basis, I would be doing everything to avoid curling up into fetal position. All I wanted to do was go home and cuddle with my puppy, Rahja.

I tried everything, including chugging half of a bottle of neon-pink Pepto-Bismol to alleviate the tight spasm in my chest, but I threw it all back up. At first, I argued with my internal doctor brain that I was at least 22 years too young for a heart attack. But I did not mess around. I went straight to my primary care doctor for help.

I traded in the La Perla for a scratchy hospital gown as I sat waiting for my doctor to arrive. She peered up at me after assessing all the facts in my flimsy medical chart. "Romie, you are like every other type A junior faculty doctor coming through here. It's just acid reflux. You gotta stop the coffee-chocolate-wine combination."

I lost my composure and gasped before catching myself. *Romie, take it like a warrior. Keep a straight face.*

"We'll start these antacids and antibiotics and send you to the GI department for additional tests."

I listened to her instructions. I stopped consuming the only three food groups that mattered to me and started the antacids and antibiotics. They didn't work, so eventually I stopped the antibiotics and restarted the chocolate; a girl has gotta cope, right? Somewhere in that period of 18 months, my overwhelmed, chronically stressed self was starting to lose the connection to the joy I used to have in seeing our epilepsy patients reach significant milestones—like going to prom, and getting a driver's license.

If you have seen my TEDx talk from 2014, you know this story. My chest pain worsened due to my chronic stress and burnout and eventually led to life-saving surgery and a forced reckoning with my lifestyle. For those of you who haven't watched the talk, *The Powerful Secret of Your Breath*, I didn't have the run-of-the-mill acid-reflux disease—which, by the way, is anything but ordinary pain. Instead, after seeing multiple specialists, including a few who thought I was making it all up in my head, and after many thorough tests from the modern-day medical world, it was a vintage test from the early 1970s—an X-ray after swallowing barium—that clued the doctors in. I had achalasia, and my biopsy wasn't clear. I now had pathology changes in my esophagus that could be early signs of something more serious (Barrett's esophagus). I didn't know what that was. I was a brain doctor. In simple terms, it meant that there was a stricture in my food pipe that was preventing me from swallowing, and the cells had morphed from a healthy lining to a toxic, possibly precancerous lesion. I ran to Dr. Google as the radiology team gave me sympathetic looks, only to find the top thirty-seven searches showing me "the rates of esophageal cancer with achalasia…" Doesn't Dr. Google always tell you that you may have cancer at your most vulnerable times? Yet even with the disabling symptoms and the fear Dr. Google had instilled in my Busy Brain, I continued to churn through each long day, and burn the midnight oil. I didn't have a choice. My schedule and to-do list multiplied even while I felt like my body was betraying me.

No matter what medication or nutrition plan I tried, nothing seemed to help the chest pain, and I found myself slipping further into a place of isolation. I would wake up in the middle of the night, completely unable to breathe, choking on my saliva and vomit. I was frequently getting sick with colds, flu, and then pneumonia. Why did my brain not come with a switch so I could turn off this overwhelming feeling?

Aside from my achalasia, modern medicine didn't have a term for my other diagnosis—my spirit was broken into pieces. I desperately wanted my disease and constant anxiety to disappear. I wanted to return to my normal of being a dutiful doctor, daughter, and doggy mama—but there was no way to stop the world from moving on without me. How was I going to keep up?

brainSCIENCE Break
Is There a Stress On-Off Switch in the Brain?

"Siri, turn off my stress, please."

"Hello, anyone?"

"Okay, it's your turn, Alexa. Turn my stress off now, dammit."

If my Aunties heard you or me bark at Siri or Alexa, they'd chime in unison, "Hai hai, yelling into your phone or some computer in the house is loud, tacky, and bad manners. This is why we still use The Clapper. You bring applause with you as you enter each room of your home."

Before the age of yelling at our smartphones and smart home devices, my Aunties were obsessed with The Clapper. For those of you who have no idea what I'm talking about, The Clapper came before artificial intelligence. You simply plugged your lamps into The Clapper before plugging them into the electrical outlet. With a clap of your hands, you could turn your lights on and off. I don't know which Auntie found the device first on some late-night home shopping network, but with one show-and-tell chai party, the trend took off, and all of our family homes were outfitted with the device. In. Every. Room. Light switches and dimmers be damned, we were going to clap our way out of darkness into seeing the light.

Wouldn't it be just wonderful to program The Clapper,

Siri, or Alexa to turn the stress off in our brains? From influencers to journalists on the evening news—everyone tries to find that one perfect stress-busting tip. Yet according to data from the American Psychology Association, Americans were stressed out, sleep-deprived, and burned out in 2019, prior to the global pandemic, and unfortunately the data continues to worsen in 2022.

I'm afraid to say, though, that even with all that wishful thinking, stress is not a feeling we can just turn off in our brains and bodies. Scrolling past one more meme suggesting that you can automatically flip a switch in your brain to "stress less and feel blessed" is misleading, especially in the face of chronic stress.

Despite all the research and advances in treatment options for stress, why are we all still overwhelmed with life, trying to find the next tip, hack, or trick to get through the rest of the workday? Our modern day work ethos expects you to either wear stress as a badge of honor or as a sign of shame that somehow you couldn't make it in the cutthroat environment known as your life.

Work-related stress remains a critical issue after the global pandemic, according to Gallup's *State of the Global Workplace 2022 Report*. Whether employees are stressed because of work, or their stress is carrying over into work, the world's employees are feeling even more stressed than they did in 2020 (the previous all-time high). Forty-four percent of employees experienced a lot of daily stress in the previous day. While almost half of the world's workers felt the burden of stress, working women in the US and Canada were among the most stressed employees globally. Stress is the underlying reason we end up in our primary care doctor's office with symptoms such as frequent colds, high blood pressure, ulcers, back pain, headaches, irregular menstrual cycles, low libido, and depression. According to the Centers for Disease Control, more than 75% of our doctors' office visits are due to these symptoms where the root cause is high stress levels or burnout.

Acute episodic and chronic stress, which we discussed in the last chapter, lead to burnout if they go unchecked and/or untreated. But stress and burnout are NOT the same, nor should the terms be interchanged. The term *burnout* was coined in the 1970s by the American psychologist Herbert Freudenberger. He used it to describe the consequences of severe stress and high ideals in "helping" professions. The World Health Organization (WHO) officially classified burnout as a "syndrome conceptualized as resulting from chronic workplace stress that has not been successfully managed," in the organization's International Classification of Diseases diagnostic manual. It is important to note that in 2019, the WHO upgraded the definition of burnout to a syndrome and added the diagnosis to the *International Classification of Diseases (ICD-11)* as an occupational phenomenon.

The three symptoms included in the diagnostic list of burnout are:

- Feelings of energy depletion or exhaustion

- Increased mental distance from one's job or negative feelings toward one's career

- Reduced professional productivity

Defining rates of burnout in the US workforce varies according to how researchers asked questions. For instance, in the *Aflac Workforces Report for 2022-23*, more than half (59%) of American workers are experiencing at least moderate levels of burnout, a notable increase over 2021 (52%) and on par with the levels reported in 2020 at the height of the COVID-19 pandemic. In this case, "moderate burnout" was defined as having one of the three symptoms defined by the WHO. Nearly 50% of employees and 53% of managers report that they're burned out at work, according to research from Microsoft, which surveyed 20,000 people in 11 countries in 2022.

In reviewing the data on stress and burnout, it's clear that no one is immune to the negative impacts of chronic stress, and the risk of developing burnout remains high.

Chronic Stress Leads to Inflammation in the Brain (and Your Body)

In the last chapter, we talked about the airport traffic control tower of your brain, known as the limbic system. Like the global airspace, your brain is connected to all the other organ systems of your body.

When we put ourselves through chronic physical, emotional, or mental stress, negative changes start to occur in the structure and function of the brain, known as neuroinflammation. Neuroinflammation is the process where the brain's own innate immune system is triggered and leads to cellular and chemical changes. In long-standing medical research spanning decades, we have known that neuroinflammation can be caused by an injury, infection, exposure to a toxin, neuro-degenerative disease, or aging in the brain.

What is really important for you (and your primary care doctors to be updated with) is that recent studies in the last decade have found that chronic stress can cause neuroinflammation too. The emotional and mental stress we perceive in our day-to-day lives is leading to neuroinflammation that we already know happens in diseases like encephalitis and dementia. To say it another way, we now know that a certain pattern of neuroinflammation can be caused by acute episodic and chronic stress. I will break down the detailed science of neuroinflammation with acute episodic and chronic stress in chapter 6. You will read more about how dangerous cytokines, specifically interleukin-1 (IL-1), are produced under chronic stress in the brain. These inflammatory markers are related to high levels of stress and anxiety disorders.

In addition to neuroinflammation raising IL-1 levels, other research shows critical markers of inflammation rise during periods of stress that primarily affect the hippocampus and prefrontal cortex of the brain.

Chronic stress can precipitate anxiety disorders and other brain health disorders such as poor memory, depression, and sleep disturbances, to name a few. How does this happen? The processing of chronic stress occurs in several pathways that link the brain and the body. The amygdala is known as the emotional processing center of the brain and was also referred to in the last chapter as the airport traffic control tower of our brain's and body's operations.

Chronic stress disrupts two key pathways in the brain: the hypothalamic-pituitary-adrenal axis, also known as the HPA axis, and the autonomic nervous system. When someone experiences a stressful event, the amygdala sends a distress signal to the hypothalamus. The hypothalamus now communicates with the rest of the body through the HPA axis and the autonomic nervous system.

The HPA axis describes the function of the interaction between the hypothalamus, pituitary gland, and adrenal glands. The main function generally attributed to the HPA axis involves the body's reaction to stress. When the HPA axis is stimulated, a myriad of stress hormones are activated, including adrenocorticotropic hormone (ACTH) and cortisol.

The hypothalamus also triggers the autonomic nervous system. The autonomic nervous system is a component of the peripheral nervous system that regulates involuntary physiologic processes, including heart rate, blood pressure, respiration, digestion, and sexual arousal. It contains three divisions: sympathetic, parasympathetic, and enteric.

When something stressful happens to us, our initial response is mediated by the sympathetic nervous system. This response occurs almost immediately and results in the secretion of epinephrine and norepinephrine, which causes symptoms like increased heart rate, elevated blood pressure, and increased perspiration.

We discussed in the last chapter that once your stress pathways are triggered through the HPA axis, the sympathetic nervous system is activated, and then the neuroinflammation pathway is triggered. We will discuss that the neuroinflammation that causes a Busy Brain is marked by the rise of pro-inflammatory cytokines in the brain that leads to neurotoxic effects. The brain and body need the counterbalancing activation of your parasympathetic nervous system to calm down the neuroinflammation.

Neuroinflammation Patterns in the Busy Brain Dysregulation of Your Circadian Rhythm

Above, we discussed how the hypothalamus is activated during chronic stress through the HPA axis. The hypothalamus also stimulates the autonomic nervous system. Also important within the hypothalamus is our internal biological clock, known as the circadian rhythm. Every organ system in our body is moderated by circadian rhythms, and they are connected to a master clock, sometimes referred to as the circadian pacemaker, located in the brain. Specifically, it is found in the suprachiasmatic nucleus (SCN), which is in a part of the hypothalamus. At different times of the day, clock genes in the SCN send signals to control activity throughout the body. One of the most important roles our circadian rhythm plays is in our sleep-wake cycle. When we are under chronic stress and have neuroinflammation, the circadian rhythm is not immune to negative impacts. This means that you have symptoms such as inability to fall asleep, low energy when you wake up in the morning, or a feeling that you are wired and tired all day long.

There is a distinct pattern of neuroinflammation that causes Busy Brain symptoms, and at the core of the problem is a disrupted circadian rhythm. You will read more in chapter 5 about the role of restoring the circadian rhythm in healing a Busy Brain. Then, in section three, you will take part in the brainSHIFT Protocol, where the first three brainSHIFTs are dedicated to helping restore our circadian rhythm.

In my story, a consistent factor that led from chronic stress to burnout was sleep deprivation. In my medical training and then my job, I was constantly "on call," meaning awake at night to take care of neurology patients in the emergency room and hospital between 5:00 p.m. and 8:00 a.m. the following morning. Some nights I was awake and walking the hospital corridors all night—trying to catch a cat nap at the ICU desk. Other nights, the minute I would put my head down on the pillow, my pager would go off to answer a phone call. Either way, I counted a period of almost 10 years when I did not get a single week of undisturbed sleep.

I look back at those years when my stress levels continued to build and eventually transitioned into burnout. I needed coffee and chocolate to keep my brain feeling rewarded to cope with my day, and then a glass of red wine at night to decompress. If I was on call and had to skip the wine, chocolate was also part of my nightly wind-down ritual. Having a Busy Brain can mean that neuroinflammation can lead to the cycle of needing caffeine in the morning for energy, and a sedative like alcohol or a sleeping pill at night.

Busy Brain: The Vicious Cycle of Anxiety, Attention Deficit Disorder (ADD), and Insomnia

As we transition from feeling chronically stressed out to burnout, a myriad of brain, mental health, and physical symptoms can appear. When I look at the pattern of chronic stress that leads to neuroinflammation and disruption of circadian rhythm, common symptoms are difficulty falling and staying asleep, and constant ruminating about worries and negative thoughts, especially before bedtime. Because of a disrupted circadian rhythm, you can experience a range of symptoms from a mild difficulty in focusing to a frank attention deficit disorder (with or without hyperactivity). As we lose focus, anxiety builds and leads to the ruminating thoughts that keep us up at night yet again. I heard about these symptoms from you too. From convention center stages to Zoom breakout rooms, listening to your stories shed light on a particular pattern that emerges when we are stuck on the stress-success cycle. I named this pattern Busy Brain.

The pattern makes us feel like our brains are spinning out of control faster than emails multiply in our inboxes. What happens when a success-driven individual feels out of control? You'll see the research results in section two of the book, showing a triad of symptoms: ruminating anxiety, difficulty focusing, and insomnia.

When I use the term *anxiety*, this can range from feelings of anxiousness to a clinical diagnosis of ruminating anxiety and/or panic attacks. Challenges in focusing during the workday can range from reduced attention span to adult-onset ADD. Insomnia presents with three distinct patterns of sleep disturbance, which we will cover in subsequent chapters.

Your Busy Brain pattern is as unique as your taste preferences for comfort food. Yet the root cause of how and why a Busy Brain occurs is similar in most adults. Here is one of many surprises the clients I work with realize once they take the Busy Brain Test. They thought functioning with anxiety, difficulty focusing, and insomnia were normal for an aging brain—or they are somehow resigned to the idea that they are a failure.

To cope with the Busy Brain, we end up on a stimulant-sedative cycle. Do you consume high amounts of caffeine and other stimulant medications to make it through your workday? By the end of the day, you need to take the edge off and want alcohol or another sedative to calm down and be present for your loved ones in the evening.

As I stood for hours (in heels) listening to these stories, I started to connect the dots, see patterns, and went back to medical journals for a scientific explanation. Too often, the first symptoms are written off as having a stressful day. This is when I coined the term *Busy Brain* to describe this specific pattern of neuroinflammation in the brain.

Let's review the symptoms of a Busy Brain again:

- You can't connect to your personality without a venti dairy-free latte in the morning. You tell me it's just coffee, but you may have added an energy drink or prescription Adderall to get going that you didn't mention.

- Your day/schedule/task list has been hijacked. There are too many browser windows open on your computer and in your brain.

- You try to focus on one important task, but the dinging of notifications to your email inbox, Slack channels, and text messages distracts you. It takes 47 minutes to finish a task that usually takes less than 3 minutes.

- You finally make it to the end of the day and need a glass of wine or bourbon to take the edge off.

- You are wired and tired—you know you will sleep well tonight, but you put your head down on your pillow and you can't shut down your racing thoughts.

- Once again, the ping of a notification pulls your finger to the screen of your phone—and you lose another 92 minutes down the Google research rabbit hole, wondering why you have been researching high-grade plungers for your bathroom.

What if I said that in our worlds of neurology and psychiatry, we missed the mark? Anxiety, adult-onset ADD, and insomnia are not three separate diseases, but all share a common root cause. The current over-the-counter treatments or prescriptions actually make this myriad of symptoms worse. Either we are using caffeine to cope during the day or alcohol at night to calm down. Or we are overprescribed stimulant medications to take during the day, such as Ritalin, and then sedated at night with prescription sleeping and anxiety medications. Either way, we are, as a society, stuck on the stimulant-sedative cycle.

We keep searching for the next fad diet or nutrition plan to give us a solution, but it feels too regimented or like a part-time job, and who has time for additional work?

No matter what protocol or treatment plan I tried for my physical symptoms, I found myself slipping further into a place of isolation. Despite being surrounded by my patients, colleagues in the hospital, and my extended family, I felt like no one saw me. Heck, I didn't recognize myself when I looked in the mirror, and avoided my own gaze. To be honest, aside from my achalasia and my Busy Brain, modern medicine didn't have a term for my other diagnosis. My spirit was broken.

When medical management of my achalasia failed, and my health continued to deteriorate, I was sent on a US tour of medical specialists in Arizona, Wisconsin, and Chicago, Illinois. They all agreed I needed urgent surgery, and the next stop on the tour was the world-renowned cardiothoracic surgery department at the University of Washington Medical Center in Seattle. I sat with my elderly parents, Daddy patting my upper arm, in the office of Dr. Carlos Pellegrini.

"You are the youngest case we have seen, and the most severe," he said.

Once again, my perfectly plotted life plan betrayed me, and I fell apart sobbing like a 4-year-old Romie who'd lost her plastic neon-red-and-yellow Fisher Price stethoscope.

Hope had officially departed my soul.

brainDUMP Chapter 2 Summary

1. Chronic stress and burnout are two different issues, and these terms should not be used interchangeably.

2. Each year, data shows that more and more workers in the US and globally report feeling stressed due to work. No one is immune to burnout.

3. Chronic stress leads to neuroinflammation, which causes elevated inflammation markers in the brain.

4. The hypothalamus is stimulated in chronic stress

through the HPA axis, leading to elevated stress hormones in the brain and the body.

5. The hypothalamus also activates the autonomic nervous system during chronic stress, specifically the sympathetic nervous system, which wreaks havoc in all the organ systems in the body.

6. Busy Brain is a specific syndrome of symptoms (anxiety, adult-onset ADD, and insomnia) that is caused by neuroinflammation disrupting the circadian rhythm.

quickSHIFT: Take Fast Action Now: What Is Your Busy Brain Score?

In fact, do you want to know if you have a Busy Brain right now? Go to the website *www.BusyBrainCure.com* and take the Busy Brain test for free. Here you will answer twenty simple questions and obtain your Busy Brain score.

In chapter 10, I'll break down the results of over 17,000 individuals who have taken the Busy Brain test since April 2020. Spoiler alert: over 80% of individuals have a score of 40, meaning that Busy Brain is leading to negative symptoms affecting mood, memory, sleep, and physical health.

3

Busy Brain Cure
One Size Does Not Fit All

I have a confession that, by now, probably won't surprise you. That day in Dr. Pellegrini's office with my parents by my side, I wore Prada. But, of course.

When I'd gotten dressed that morning, I heard the Aunties in my head: *Ooouffff, no one will give you bad news today if you are dressed up like you are going to a wedding. Plus, you never know, you may meet a handsome SINGLE doctor. Put on jasmine perfume and your Nanni's ruby ring as a blessing.*

When I'd stepped out of the bathroom in the hotel room in Seattle, adorned in my outfit of the day, my parents carefully surveyed the situation, then glanced at each other in a daze of confusion. My mother then looked at my father and said, "What is happening in the next chapter of the drama known as our daughter?"

Daddy approached me cautiously, eyeing the black-and-white-print cocktail dress and sandals. "Baytuh, we are going to the surgeon's office today, right? So, why do you look like you are dressed for a fancy dinner party in New York City?"

"No one is going to tell me today that I am dying. I am wearing couture." My answer to my father may have been my desi-girl version of executing fake it till you make it, but inside I was sinking in a cesspool of fear.

"Thohba, thohba, thohba." He knew better than to argue with the ancient wisdom of my judgmental Aunties.

But later in the surgeon's office, when Dr. Pellegrini said, "You are the youngest case we have seen, and the most severe," I broke down sobbing, in deep pain, and Daddy tried desperately to comfort me.

Dr. Pellegrini continued, "We are going to start with one surgery and operate on your lower esophagus and stomach, but you will likely need one to two more operations in the next 18 months. If the biopsy finds cancer, do you want to continue the treatment here in Seattle or near your parents' home?" He paused, and added, "Do you have disability insurance?"

Snot ran down my face, and I didn't need my MAC compact to know that my eyes were bloodshot. I'd been in Dr. Pellegrini's seat delivering similar news to patients, but on this side of the desk, I didn't know how to process his words. Instead, I puked all over my Prada.

To the patron saints of fashion and to all the fash-un queens reading (or listening), please accept my repentance. Hands-On-My-Chanel-Purse, I now understand that vomit belongs in the wastebasket or toilet.

But honestly, have you ever been in a position where your perfectly curated life was suddenly raw and exposed? In public? I'm sure you too have suffered some variation of a puke-on-your-Prada moment. We go to college and climb the ladders of success, yet no one has created a warning label for life stating that living a chronically stressed-out life can be dangerous for your health and your perfectly curated wardrobe. (Until now, that is.)

And to whoever started the mantra "fake it till you make it": here, hold my trash can.

brainSCIENCE Break

When our health and thus our lives are falling apart, the last thing our brains can process is where to start looking for help. Navigating the wellness marketplace and searching for the right cure for chronic stress and a Busy Brain can be as confusing and expensive as curating a designer capsule wardrobe.

Well-meaning coworkers and friends (or judgmental Aunties) all think they have the perfect solution, usually found through a social media influencer. You might even try it, but it doesn't work for you. Maybe you consider going to your primary care doctor, but you're afraid of hearing bad news or being given a prescription medicine with a slew of side effects. Instead, maybe you just look on Dr. Google, but find that the algorithm offers little help or hope but does offer you up recommendations based on your past search results. In my case, searching for "self-care for stress relief" brings up shoe sales.

The Continuum of Chronic Stress, Busy Brain, and Burnout

In the last chapter, I started to discuss the problem that we interchange the words *stress* and *burnout*. A Busy Brain is one pathway that can lead to a health or life disaster.

As a simple reminder, when we're stressed, if we have the luxury to "get away" from the stressor to rest or to take a vacation, we feel improvement in our mood and symptoms. However, continued acute episodic and chronic stress can lead to a Busy Brain, and if a Busy Brain goes untreated, it can eventually lead to burnout. Once we get to burnout, a Busy Brain may persist, but we likely shift from wired and tired to a place of low energy and despair.

When I transitioned from the role of doctor to patient and puked on my Prada that day, the term "burnout" wasn't used or recognized in society, let alone in medicine. Sitting between my parents, I couldn't shake the feeling that somehow I had failed. I simply couldn't cut it in the world of traditional cut-throat academic medicine. Eventually, I would even be guided by my father and uncles, all of whom were doctors, to suck it up, and change the type of medical job I worked in. We all had the assumption that if I went to a community hospital setting, I would be back on track. We told ourselves that in the community setting, I would have fewer demands than in an academic medical center; I would only have to see patients and not have the pressure to do research, publish journal articles, and teach medical students. But in fact, it never works to jump from one hamster wheel to another—regardless of what type of shoes you are wearing.

That's the problem when we have a Busy Brain or are burned out; we may think the quick fix is to change jobs, wardrobes, spouses, houses, or the cities where we live. When we are stuck on the stress-success cycle, our minds trick us into thinking if we can just achieve one more goal, our stress and worries will disappear. But…if we don't get to the root cause of our Busy Brain, guess what? The stressors of change and a new job/career/marriage will continue to fuel our Busy Brains and can lead to burnout.

You can see through my story that what started with the best of intentions—to succeed at all costs—led to stress. Early in my career, if I could catch up on sleep without a night on call for the hospital, I would feel re-energized. But as my stress continued, I started to have difficulty focusing and felt anxious. Eventually, my job and stress deprived me of so much sleep that I couldn't catch up. I started to depend on coffee-chocolate-wine to get through my day. Over time, as the responsibilities, deadlines, and my health issues piled on, I started to slip into that dark place. As my Busy Brain and achalasia symptoms worsened, I lost the passion and joy for a job I loved. By the time I ended up in surgery, I had slipped further into an unexplained darkness. We now know that darkness is burnout.

Unlike stress, where you can imagine feeling better once things settle, burnout feels hopeless. Burnout is a cycle of negative emotions and withdrawal that results from investing too much into something emotionally, intellectually, or physically without doing anything to restore yourself.

The American Psychological Association (APA) has surveyed adults in the United States annually since 2007 to assess stress levels. To no one's surprise, the numbers worsen yearly. The data for 2022, the most recent data available at the publication of this book, showed that stress in adults in the United States is negatively impacting every aspect of our health:

Seventy-six percent of adults reported they had experienced at least one symptom in the last month as a result of stress. What were these symptoms?

- Headache (38%)

- Fatigue (35%)

- Feeling nervous or anxious (34%)

- Feeling depressed or sad (33%)

Seven in ten adults (72%) experienced additional symptoms in the last month, and the most common symptoms reported were

- Feeling overwhelmed (33%)

- Experiencing changes in sleeping habits (32%)

- Constantly worrying (30%).

When directly asked about the relationship between stress and jobs, American workers exhibited high rates of at least one symptom of burnout. According to the APA's *2021 Work and Well-being Survey* of 1,501 US adult workers,

- Seventy-nine percent of employees had experienced work-related stress in the month before the survey.

- Nearly three in five employees reported negative impacts of work-related stress, including lack of interest, motivation, or energy (26%) and lack of effort at work (19%).

- Meanwhile, 36% reported cognitive weariness, 32% reported emotional exhaustion, and an astounding 44% reported physical fatigue—a 38% increase since 2019.

In these reports, teachers and healthcare workers have higher rates of burnout symptoms compared to other professions, but let us be clear. No one is immune. Since I shared my story of burnout publicly in my TEDx talk in 2014, I have been invited to speak at over 550 in-person and virtual lectures in every industry—from the technology sector to education to finance to hospitality. As I said, no one is immune to the negative impacts of stress on their brain and body. If your particular symptoms of stress have led you to lose focus, feel anxious, and have difficulty falling and staying asleep, then I welcome you to join us to cure your Busy Brain.

In early 2020, when many sectors sent their employees home to work remotely, our business model of speaking and consulting also had to adapt to use technology. The benefit of speaking to teams using Zoom was being able to give the Busy Brain Test online instead of virtually. The Busy Brain Test is a validated neuropsychology test that measures how stress affects your health. (You can take the Busy Brain Test for free at *www.BusyBrainCure.com*.) Between June 1, 2020, and December 2022, about 17,000 people took the test online, and 83% of people had a score above 40, indicating their stress symptoms were leading toward burnout. What were the most common symptoms reported in the Busy Brain Test results from 2020 through 2022? Difficulty falling asleep, waking up in the middle of the night and being unable to fall back asleep, and maintaining energy during the day. Sound familiar?

The Busy Brain Test is a previously validated neuropsychology test that consists of twenty questions, which assess the effects of stress in four key areas:

1. Sleep

2. Daytime energy and focus

3. Mental health

4. Physical/hormonal symptoms

Are you wondering what your score is on the Busy Brain Test? At the end of the last chapter, I offered you the opportunity to take the Busy Brain Test to obtain your score. Did you score above a 30? Did you realize that some of the symptoms you are experiencing may be related to stress or even burnout? If you didn't get your score in the last chapter, you can go to the link (*www.BusyBrainCure.com*) and take 3 minutes to answer twenty questions.

One-Size Solutions Don't Fit All Busy Brains

In the world of couture clothing, if the fit is not correct, you become a fashion fail. In the world of traditional medicine, we often treat disease management with a one-cure-fits-all mentality. Like the dress or suit you last wore, one size does not fit all. Hell, it may not even fit *you* the week before your period. Looking for a solution for your stress and Busy Brain is no different. We cannot prescribe the exact same protocol to every person. As I mentioned in the last chapter, the symptoms of a Busy Brain are ruminating anxiety, difficulty focusing or adult-onset attention deficit disorder, and insomnia. When you look at the traditional medical management of each of these symptoms, it involves the same classes of medications—either stimulants or sedatives. We also talked about being stuck on the stimulant-sedative cycle in the last chapter. Don't get me wrong. If only one of those symptoms is present, a prescription medication may be in order. But have you ever wondered, am I just using a Band-Aid rather than fixing the problem? Oftentimes with prescription medication, you are.

The current mainstream medications for anxiety are not completely effective for most of the population, their side effects outweigh potential benefits, or they are addicting.

One class of medications used for generalized anxiety disorder is the benzodiazepines, such as lorazepam and clonazepam. In a large meta-analysis review of benzodiazepines published in *Lancet* in 2019, this class of drugs was found to be highly effective in reduction of anxiety and associated symptoms for generalized anxiety disorders (GAD) in the acute setting. Generally, they lead to a reduction of symptoms within minutes to hours depending on the specific medication. However, there is a potential for abuse and dependence on benzodiazepines, and some of these medications can actually cause rebound anxiety. Rebound anxiety means that after a temporary treatment or calming of anxiety symptoms, they return with a vengeance. What first worked to treat the anxiety may no longer work, and the symptoms may be even more severe. A side effect of this class of medications is sedation, which reduces daytime energy and ability to focus. Typically, these medications are supposed to be prescribed by physicians in an emergency setting or after other options have been tried and failed.

Another class of medications that is commonly prescribed by physicians for anxiety disorders is known as the selective serotonin reuptake inhibitors (SSRIs), such as fluoxetine and citalopram. A large systematic review in *Psychotherapy and Psychosomatics Journal* in 2013 shows these medications are more effective in treating anxiety that exists with depression, but have little efficacy in treating generalized anxiety disorders. In a research study published in *Journal of Consulting and Clinical Psychology* in 2016, Dr. Christopher Rosnick and colleagues assessed serum cortisol levels (stress hormone) in adults with anxiety. They found that participants had lower cortisol levels and improved treatment of anxiety if you combined cognitive behavioral therapy with an SSRI medication, compared to just the medication alone. Bottom line, both studies found that approximately 50 to 60% of people saw improvement in anxiety scores and felt better, but unfortunately for up to 40% of these patients, they had a relapse of anxiety.

The sedative prescription medications typically used to treat insomnia are also sedating and are grouped in categories called benzodiazepine receptor agonists and non-benzodiazepine insomnia medications. Examples of these medications that you see advertised on television in the US all too often are zolpidem and temazepam. Again, the potential for dependency runs deep in these medications, and they are only supposed to be used temporarily for up to 14 days. In a large systemic review of these medications published in the *Journal of General Internal Medicine* in 2007, these medications were found to be effective in helping you fall asleep quickly and stay asleep. Pitfalls of these medications include dependency and limiting you from reaching deeper stages of sleep needed for a complete sense of rest.

I am not against prescription medicines. However, I wonder if the medication we are prescribing is treating your symptoms or actually treating the underlying cause of a Busy Brain. Haven't you ever wondered, why did I develop these symptoms? Is there something deeper going on that we are missing? What is actually at the root of why the symptoms started, continued, and are now hijacking my sense of control?

Finding a Root Cause

In integrative medicine, physicians use science-backed research to understand how to get to the root cause of your symptoms. Integrative medicine uses an evidence-based approach to treat the whole person—mind, body, and soul. Don't cue the crystal singing bowls or start burning sage around this book. Integrative medicine is the future, even if it's not wholly integrated in the medical model right now. But read this with emphasis: your physical, emotional, mental, and spiritual needs are all involved in your health, so integrative medicine uses a combination of therapies. It "integrates" conventional approaches (surgery and medications) and complementary therapies (yoga, acupuncture, nutrition, meditation, etc.) to achieve optimal health and healing.

Don't misinterpret my love for traditional medicine, but

do know that on my journey to healing from achalasia, the answers came through traditional medications, life-saving surgery, AND complementary therapies found in integrative medicine. I was blessed that the biopsy did not show cancerous lesions, but we didn't have an answer as to why my achalasia symptoms were so severe. The doctors did the corrective surgery on my esophagus and stomach, but as I lay in the hospital afterward, the one question that plagued me was, Now, how do I fix the rest of my life? I still had not found a way to take control of my Busy Brain. I felt so lost and no longer had a road map to my perfectly plotted existence. I couldn't help feeling that nothing I had learned in medical school was going to help me now.

brainDUMP Chapter 3 Summary

• Episodic and chronic stress can lead to Busy Brain symptoms.

• In our research, 83% of people who took the Busy Brain Test had symptoms that stress was negatively impacting their health or that they were already burned out.

• There is no one-size-fits-all outfit that is fashionable or functional for all—the same goes for medications and treatments.

• Current treatments for anxiety and insomnia have the potential for side effects and are only a Band-Aid for your symptoms.

- Integrative medicine uses scientific research to treat the whole person—mind, body, and spirit—while getting to the root cause of your disease.

quickSHIFT: Medicine Cabinet Check

How many prescription medication bottles, supplements, and other random gadgets do you have in your home that you have tried using for insomnia, anxiety, and improving your attention? When I have worked with clients one-on-one or in our brainSHIFT 8-week group program, individuals often can't remember what they have tried to help Busy Brain symptoms, or forgot something was on the shelf.

Could you make a list of the following items?

1. The medications and supplements you are currently taking for sleep, anxiety, focus/attention (Busy Brain).

2. Prescription medications you have tried for sleep, anxiety, or focus/attention in the past.

3. Over-the-counter medications you have tried for Busy Brain in the past.

4. Supplements you have tried in the past.

5. Smartphone applications, online programs, or other technology you have tried using or are currently using.

The goal of this exercise is not only to help you organize your medications and supplements, but also to create an outline and history of your journey that will be helpful when you start the brainSHIFT Protocol in section three of this book. Trust me, it's annoying to go to the doctor for answers, only to find that you forgot you tried that medication or supplement before. Another sign of a Busy Brain is that the expired supplement bottles are jammed behind your collection of face creams or stacked in the mix of all of your flavored protein shakes.

4

How Do You Cure a Busy Brain?

I want to take you back 4 years before my achalasia symptoms began to show you how I fell from grace in my perfectly plotted life. I sat in a tailored pantsuit and focused on the welcome/initiation speech by one of my male physician colleagues where I had my first attending neurology position (my first grown-up medical job).

The speech went like this: "Dr. Mushtaq, you are not planning to get pregnant, are you? The other woman in the department had complications with her pregnancy and was out for almost 6 months. The department lost over a million dollars in revenue. We need you to work like a man."

Forget the fact that I was divorced and had been single for 2 years or that I was the sole breadwinner in my household. The blatant sexism in the patriarchal world of medicine reminded me yet again that the glass ceiling was not only present, but suffocating. I got the memo loud and clear. If you are going to survive, you are selling your soul to the healthcare system. Any semblance of a personal goal or desires outside of work should immediately cease.

I'd entered neurology at a time when less than 5% of brain doctors in the United States were women. I desperately tried to keep my head down, my heels high, and stay laser-focused on work. But underneath the starched white lab coat, I was trying to hide a carefully curated secret. My brain and body were struggling to keep up with the demands of my work and my pushing for success at all costs. But no one told me the cost would be my career and life as I knew it.

Fast forward 4 years into my work in that same department and my achalasia symptoms were raging. That man's speech was still on loop in my Busy Brain, haunting me all these years later. My Jimmy Choos clicked across sterile tiles without their usual sense of confidence. My head hung down, and my long frizzy hair half covered my face. This was my doctor version of a walk of shame—I'd let my personal stuff (read: debilitating illness) affect my work, as hard as I'd tried not to. I'd spent the previous night in an unromantic rendezvous with my pager while vomiting up anything I was trying to eat or drink. I was coming off a long call night on the neurology floor, and now I was rounding in the neurology unit for the last time before I left my academic job for the hopefully easier community hospital job. The irony and pain. I was not pregnant (pregnancy wasn't even an option in my body—I had tried and failed at that too). So, I had fulfilled that portion of the missive, but we were beginning to work up the diagnosis and treatment of my achalasia at this point, and I had to take my soul out of the healthcare system for a time.

To this day, I remember my patients, even their parents or spouses who accompanied them, asking me often, "Doc, are you okay? Are you taking care of yourself?" during some of the worst days of my symptoms. But as I dutifully answered every page and completed every consult, not a single physician colleague looked me in the eye or asked if I was okay, even while I was choking on my saliva or coming to work with pneumonia. They were happy to discuss a clinical case or drone on about last night's game on ESPN. They noticed something was off, all right, don't get me wrong. The nursing staff, EEG technicians, and administrators were all too happy to pass on the gossip to me, the comments about how "that's what happens when you let a woman into the academy." In the toxic work culture of clinical medicine, you either shut up and keep up, or you are labeled weak and not worthy of your MD credentials. To admit to anyone the actual truth that I was in need of medical leave would have been the end of my career, because this was a concept that was not allowed in academic medicine at that time. Vacations were used only in the case of a family emergency, and really, what is a family emergency when you are not allowed a personal life? We won't even get into the subject of how I had to pay to see my therapist out of pocket and use a fake name so that the visit wouldn't be tracked on my health insurance bill. Seeking professional mental health help could lead to loss of a doctor's credentialing and licensing.

When I returned to my parents' home after surgery to recover, the real Aunties (not the ones in my mind) visited me daily, and I heard, "What happened to the Romie we knew? You were so happy as a little girl here in this home reading encyclopedias and eating chocolate. I look at you now and it is as if the lights are on, but nobody is home."

If that was their diagnosis, I was suffering in the stillness. I was forced to lie still for a long time, both in that hospital bed in Seattle and in my parents' home afterward. My body and my bruised spirit needed time to heal and recover. In that silence, a loud jerk showed up in my mind with a firm voice of judgment and condemnation.

You are a failure. You failed your parents and brought shame to your elders and ancestors. You failed all women in medicine.

I did not know how to shut down these condemning voices in my head.

Little did I know that in the ancient herbal tea recipes, the murghi ka shorba (now sold in the US as chicken bone broth), and the meditation cassette tapes the Aunties brought, I would find the start of a new road map—one that led to healing my body and my spirit. As I meditated, I noticed my postoperative chest pain feeling better, and I didn't need as many pain medications.

"Ah, there is our little Romie coming back to us..." my Aunties said as they continued to sit by my side, feeding me, caressing me, or fervently praying over me—sometimes a combination of all three.

I also noticed that the darkness that had a grasp on my spirit was letting go, and some—but not all—of the jerk voices were quieting down. Was it really catching up on sleep, meditating, and eating healthy traditional foods? That question sent me on a worldwide journey, where I learned about meditation and mindfulness from monks and yoga teachers. Back then, this was abnormal and weird behavior for a doctor, so

I shamefully hid the fact that I found peace of mind with my pranayama teacher in Bali or yoga therapist in Arizona. I also learned about other global healing traditions that pre-date the Western philosophy of medicine, such as Ayurveda, the ancient traditional Indian medicine dating over 5,000 years. I returned home, realizing not only was I on the journey of my own healing but that I needed to bring mindfulness and integrative medicine into helping my patients.

As I recovered from surgery and found a path to mindfulness and healing through integrative medicine, I started to gain clarity. I wasn't put through this ordeal to lose hope and beat myself up for not achieving the life goals I had mapped out since I was a child (with the careful editing of my Aunties). If I had found a way to succeed without stressing myself out (most days) and had broken the stimulant-sedative cycle, I needed to share this information with my patients. To be honest, at that time, in traditional medicine, I was seen as an outcast. In many neurology circles, I still am a source of shame and bewilderment. I spent a year shining in my fellowship training marked as the next academic research superstar in neurology by one of my previous mentors, and then contact ceased when I left my position to have my surgery. Years later, at a colleague's daughter's traditional Southern wedding, he broke all social protocol by ignoring me when I said hello. His wife only addressed me to ask for the name of my plastic surgeon that completed my boob job. To be clear, my chest size is no one's business, but it is naturally inherited by my Punjabi Aunties. In the Punjabi culture, we celebrate curves as much as comfort food.

In 2012, my colleagues in the hospital heard that I was

checking an extensive laboratory evaluation for my neurology patients to look for the root causes of headaches, depression, and other brain health issues. These were evaluations not typically performed in those days in traditional medicine. I was also teaching patients suffering from anxiety about different meditation and pranayama techniques. Most of the time, I found that the hospital-allotted time of 15 to 30 minutes in the office was not enough to create a full plan to heal mind, body, and spirit. (That time is about 5 minutes now.)

The Aunties had correctly diagnosed the aspect of burnout I could not see for myself: "It is as if the lights are on, but nobody is home." I didn't know at the time that the jerk in my mind was related to my postoperative chest pain and a myriad of other symptoms related to my belly, hormones, and sleep. I noticed my usually chattering Aunties soften up on their approach with me—both in person and in my head. I wanted to know, why did I feel a euphoria when completing a hatha yoga class? In savasana, I could hear an inner voice of knowledge, comfort, and wisdom. Where was this coming from? The rational neurologist in me needed answers. It wasn't until I started to read more and pursue my fellowship in integrative medicine that I learned about an important aspect of the mind-body connection. When the mind is at peace, the body heals. When the mind is stuck in a Busy Brain, the body starts to develop disease.

In 2014, I transitioned from traditional neurology to join an outpatient concierge integrative medicine clinic in Orlando, Florida. I now had 90 minutes with each patient and could do a full assessment of their whole life. The results from the protocol that I had begun using were transformative, but I knew I had three problems.

Problem 1: I could only reach the people who could afford to pay our high fees. I was taught by my parents and extended family about service-minded leadership, meaning to always give back. Yet I felt like I was failing, because seeing an integrative medicine physician was and is expensive, affordable to only a select few. Treating only the 1% of the 1% of society who had this type of expendable cash limited me from being of service to more people.

Problem 2: I could only see five to six people a day; how could I scale this solution? More importantly, how would I get this message out to people before their stress and burnout took over, and they ended up on a health journey similar to mine?

Problem 3: By the time patients reach an integrative medicine doctor, they have already been on the path of stress, a Busy Brain, and burnout. What if I could go to the source—our workplaces—and start a conversation with leaders? Something along the lines of, "Hey, corporate leaders, don't let the job kill you or your employees!" The reality of the workplace today is that change is happening at a pace more rapid than the human psyche is accustomed to dealing with. Because of our dependency on digital devices, there are no longer boundaries for our brains between work and our personal lives. All of these factors can and will increase our stress levels and fuel a Busy Brain.

brainSCIENCE Break

Do you have a jerk (or voices of your judgmental family members) who comes to visit and take over your mind from time to time? Are you thinking about the failures in your life, wearing them as a badge of dishonor? As we progress through chronic stress, a Busy Brain, and potentially burnout, the judgy voices, negative thoughts, or sense of hopelessness can heighten.

The treatment to recovery time from the diagnosis of my achalasia was about 18 months. The journey to correctly diagnose and heal my Busy Brain and burnout took a lot longer; I honestly didn't keep a timeline. I will tell you this: the journey I'm taking you on to understand and cure your Busy Brain took me over 16 years in my career as a doctor, researcher, patient, healer, and now founder of the brainSHIFT Institute. Today we take brain science and mental health programs to teach workplace wellness and culture to companies around the world. In 2018 I was named Chief Wellness Officer at Evolution Hospitality. At that time, over 7,000 employees worked in over 125 hotels we managed in the United States and Canada. My role was to help create and implement strategy for a mindfulness and wellness program for the organization.

What Is the Cure for Your Busy Brain in a Busy World?

The problem is not our busy schedules but how our brain processes tasks, emotions, memories, and incoming information 24/7. I researched and created the brainSHIFT Protocol to help you jump off the stress-success cycle and cure your Busy Brain.

Is there really a cure? Yes. (Or I wouldn't be writing this book and traveling over 150,000 domestic US miles a year to speak and consult with the companies and organizations where you work.) The truth is, when we cure our Busy Brains, we create a shift, what I call a brainSHIFT, that helps us do the following:

1. Choose to be productive instead of busy.

2. Replace the dopamine high of checking off to-do list items with focused intention on one project at a time.

3. Be present in the role that is required of us in the present moment.

4. Heal the neuroinflammation in our brains so we can alleviate the negative impact of stress on our health.

5. Restore the balance and diurnal variation of circadian rhythm to feel energized during the day and welcome peaceful sleep at night.

The Busy Brain Cure Is Individualized for You and Scaled for Teams

Being on the stress-success cycle keeps you in constant motion, seeking the dopamine high of crossing off the next item on your to-do list or using the adrenaline from a tight deadline to push you through the day. All the while, another stress hormone known as cortisol rises in the brain and body. This is the foundation of the neurochemistry in the Busy Brain that I will discuss in the next section of the book.

This neurochemical process accounts for the following symptoms of a Busy Brain:

1. The lack of energy in the morning and the inability to focus are adult-onset attention deficit disorders.

2. This low-level feeling of anxiousness builds to ruminating anxiety, which compounds the ADD to kill productivity.

3. The symptoms bleed into your evening and lead to patterns of sleep disruption.

In a world of conflicting health advice, how can we (the professionals cursed with a Busy Brain) find a cure without forcing our clients to go on another diet? You will read in section two, chapter 8, that in brainSHIFT, the word *diet* is a four-letter curse word. The diet industry alone has disrupted our mental health, our family meals, and even what we see on social media. We created a plan that not only allows but celebrates eating comfort food. In the next section, you will learn the difference between comfort and stress eating. The number one question and source of confusion I get from our associates at Evolution Hospitality, where I serve as Chief Wellness Officer, revolves around the latest myth or food trend. Yet when we look at our workforces and collective circle of loved ones, no two nutrition plans are the same. At brainSHIFT Institute, we celebrate diversity, equity, inclusion, and belonging. And in the South Asian household where I was raised, food was a love language. One of my big goals is to create a healthier world where vegans, paleo followers, intermittent fasters, and chocolate lovers can all eat at one table—in peace.

In order to create the cure for your Busy Brain, I combined my over 20 years of experience as a doctor and researcher. I brought together my worlds of neurology and integrative medicine and added a dash of soul and sass (inherited from my Aunties, obviously). I thought back to all the individual patients I treated in neurology and integrative medicine with similar symptoms—and had to plan. How do we scale this concept to share it with teams and the public at large? For the last 3 years, I've been implementing and researching the brainSHIFT Protocol with individuals and teams in corporate America. In this book, you are going to hear the stories of individuals, teams, and organizations who completed the 8-week plan that I will walk you through.

The brainSHIFT Protocol is our program that we tested and refined online with over 1,000 executives completing the program. Okay, I know, I know, I am starting to sound like my rambling Aunties. I can hear your Busy Brain screaming at the book, "Now get to the point!"

Psycho-Neuro-Immuno-Endocrinology: The Foundation of the Busy Brain Cure

My next series of failures—I mean, experiments—to keep my Busy Brain occupied happened in recovery when I tried to find a hobby. A hobby was a luxury I didn't have as a professor in neurology. I have had challenges with hobbies that stick and would consider myself a hobby hoarder—I attempted dozens of things, but none lasted more than 30 days. For example, my attempt at gardening was over in less than 3 days when, in an attempt to plant petunias that remind me of my mother's summertime joy, I ended up with anthills and dead flowers. The only thing I knew how to do consistently that I enjoyed was reading nonfiction books—research in brain science, mental health, and holistic medicine.

Today, as a self-described geek girl, I have one desire if I had free time. My hobby would be to return to obtain a PhD in psycho-neuro-immuno-endocrinology. (By the way, now you know why I am awkward if you have ever met me on a first date or at your company's cocktail reception.) Psycho-neuro-immuno-endocrinology explains how the mind and body are connected, and it studies the interaction between the psyche, neural function of brain cells, endocrine function, and immune responses.

The four components of psycho-neuro-immuno-endocrinology are as follows:

1. *Psyche* is your mood and emotional processing of external events.

2. *Neuro* refers to the structure and function of your brain.

3. *Immuno* regards how your immune system reacts to the environment created by your mood and brain function.

4. *Endocrinology* is the study of hormones, and in psycho-neuro-immuno-endocrinology specifically, how the

hormone axis from the brain to the body reacts to changes in our external environment.

In simple terms, psycho-neuro-immuno-endocrinology means that your mood affects the function of your brain, immune system, gut health, and hormones.

Epigenetic factors and chronic stress from different types of stimuli acting through distinct pathways and neurotransmitters are highly involved in altering your psycho-neuro-immuno-endocrine axis, and this results in the onset and worsening of diseases. So the bottom line is that when chronic stress or burnout activates the psycho-neuro-immuno-endocrinology system, we trigger a myriad of symptoms in our brains and every organ system in our body. In section two, you are going to learn more about the specific patterns of neuroinflammation that are associated with the symptoms of a Busy Brain. In section three, you will be introduced to the 8-week brainSHIFT Protocol to help cure your Busy Brain by addressing all the key aspects of the psycho-neuro-immuno-endocrinology system.

What Is a brainSHIFT? Key Microhabits to Shift the Busy Brain

We cannot rebuild our relationships or businesses without getting the state of our brains straight. We get our brains straight through one action—brainSHIFT.

Breaking down brainSHIFT

The brainSHIFT Protocol is our proprietary and researched series of sustainable microhabits that heal burnout and cure Busy Brain. A microhabit is one simple, easy-to-execute habit to improve your health and well-being that feels natural and joyful for you to implement. When we master one microhabit, we then stack on the next microhabit. Habit stacking helps you add one microhabit to the next in an order that naturally builds upon one another.

New York Times bestselling author James Clear explains why microhabits work in his book, *Atomic Habits*. He explains that habits are a compound interest in self-improvement. If you want better results, then forget about setting goals. Focus on your system instead. Success is the product of daily habits— not once-in-a-lifetime transformations.

When we brainSHIFT, we do not allow the jerk in our minds to stop us before we get started, but instead, we focus on one microhabit at a time. The 8-week program is designed to try by yourself, as I did with hundreds of individual patients and coaching clients since 2013. However, we also wanted to create a free online community, or invite your team at work to complete this protocol together. As Clear discusses, "We tend to imitate the habits of three social groups: the close (family and friends), the many (the tribe), and the powerful (those with status and prestige)... One of the most effective things you can do to build better habits is to join a culture where (1) your desired behavior is the normal behavior and (2) you already have something in common with the group."

You'll read transformational stories of our clients and teams in section three of this book, but all of them had one thing in common. They committed to the 8-week program as individuals in our clinic practice, as a group in an online community, or with their team at work, where we used the concept of microhabits and tied it into cohort-based learning. You can complete the protocol in this book by yourself, but I don't want you to feel socially isolated during your transformation. It is why we created a free online community that you can access by going to the website: *www.BusyBrainCure.com*.

Cohort-based learning is a collaborative approach to learning in which students or individuals advance together throughout a course, program, or project. Instructors or mentors lead the group of students to complete given milestones. Students, either in person or online, foster a community within the group by learning together, providing social support, and collaborating. Depending on the course design, there may be an overarching goal for the entire cohort or individual goals for each student set by the instructor.

Psychology studies show that if we want to adapt a change in our health and wellness, we are more likely to succeed in the company of others. To put it a different way, how many times have you had the best intentions to put into practice what you read in these self-help books, yet you go back to your old habits? You are not alone. This is why we created the brainSHIFT Protocol for teams and have an application where you can join my team leading the protocol for our global community virtually.

As I mentioned, the brainSHIFT 8-week program is comprised of weekly microhabits that build upon each other to cure your Busy Brain. When you brainSHIFT, you can begin your day feeling energized, focused, and calm. And when you come home, you can easily switch out of work mode and shift into calm consciousness so that you may be present in your personal life. The brainSHIFT Protocol is designed to optimize your well-being in three key areas:

1. VITALITY: boost daytime energy and your ability to focus.

2. RESTORATION: restore sleep and sanity.

3. SENSE OF BELONGING: feel connected to life purpose and promote teamwork while boosting morale.

How did I pick the microhabits to improve or cure your Busy Brain? The microhabits in the brainSHIFT Protocol were researched, tested, and repeated. I wanted to find the most impactful microhabits that fit the following criteria:

1. Would result in immediate improvement in sleep.

2. Can help to boost daytime energy and focus.

3. Get to the root cause of your Busy Brain, which may be different than someone else's Busy Brain.

4. Make it fun and scalable to present to teams as a wellness program.

5. Make sure we were not stuck on another diet.

The brainSHIFT Protocol was created after years of testing in the field and keeping up with the latest medical research. The "SHIFT" in brainSHIFT is an acronym for the five key areas that are responsible for the root cause of Busy Brain in most individuals. I will break down each of the five key areas of disruption of a Busy Brain in section two of this book. Every Busy Brain is unique, and together we will figure out the root cause of your Busy Brain.

As I furthered my studies of mindfulness, meditation, and yoga, I grappled with the same issues as many of you. I didn't want to be told to slow down and go with the flow. I am and always will be an unapologetic, success-driven, type A professional. The men and women in our global brainSHIFT community share the same ethos. We are the change-makers, leaders, parents, caregivers, philanthropists, go-getters, and doers of our communities. What is the secret to breaking the stress-success cycle? Is it possible to be in all those roles and achieve your goals without getting a Busy Brain?

I wanted to take the protocol that helped me heal after surgery and share it in an accessible way so that more people could heal their Busy Brains. In the next two sections of the book, you will hear the stories of individuals and corporate teams who joined the brainSHIFT movement. Long before workplace wellness programs and mindfulness apps were on trend, these individuals and teams had the courage and the vision to say, "We know our company/industry/organization's transition period is stressful; we want to help heal stress and optimize our people's performance."

If you had asked me in that moment in the hospital bed after surgery, would I envision myself here, writing this book for you? No. I took it one day at a time to come out of it, just as it took one day at a time for years to end up with a Busy

Brain and then burnout. There is no quick fix, but it doesn't have to take you years of trial and error. I learned two things during my time of healing. I had to make the conscious decision to heal rather than play victim to the larger system of broken operations that led to my burnout. I also had to realize that I needed to step out of my comfort zone and try new ideas and solutions.

In the third section of this book, I will introduce the cure for your Busy Brain, the 8-week brainSHIFT Protocol. brainSHIFT is founded on these two principles above: holistic healing based in science and cohort-based learning—going through the program with a community.

I look back at my 20-year journey that started with medical school and progressed through internship, residency, two fellowships, and then as a practicing neurologist. While I was surrounded by classmates and colleagues, the battle to succeed while wearing stress as a badge of honor left me feeling isolated, lonely, and often without hope. When I shifted my life's path to integrative medicine and entrepreneurship, my intention for every client interaction and program was to foster a sense of caring, compassion, and community.

Like an Auntie opening up her formal living room, replete with an old wedding quilt draped over the sofa, to an esteemed guest—you—I invite you to brainSHIFT.

brainDUMP Chapter 4 Summary

1. There are solutions in both Western medicine and global healing traditions. You should not be made to pick one over the other.

2. Don't go down the healing road alone. Whether I was in a room of like-minded individuals meditating in silence or hearing the loud judgments (wisdom) of well-meaning Aunties, a sense of community heals the spirit.

3. What is a brainSHIFT? Key microhabits that stack weekly to help cure the Busy Brain.

4. The brainSHIFT Protocol is an 8-week program (preferably done in community) that restores sleep, sanity, and a sense of connection. We have created a free community of other people with Busy Brains reading this book. You can join it at *www. BusyBrainCure.com*.

quickSHIFT: Are the Lights On, but Nobody Is Home?

We are a global family, albeit one that disagrees. But do me one favor.

Do you avoid your gaze in the mirror when you are brushing your teeth in the morning? (I hope you brushed your teeth—don't let a Busy Brain drive you to your laptop in the morning without hygiene.) Or is a colleague avoiding your gaze in the office or video conference call?

Can you do one thing this week for me? Find that colleague and let them know you care. Are you unsure of what to say?

How about, "Hi, friend, it's me, Romie. I want you to know I am here for you and I care."

And if you forgot to brush your teeth, go back. Look in the mirror and tell yourself, "Hello, I am here for you, and I care for you. You got this."

SECTION TWO

The Scientific Cause of Your
Busy Brain
and the BrainSHIFT Acronym

5

Sleep and the Circadian Rhythm of a Busy Brain

The suffering of Cambodia has been deep.
From this suffering comes Great Compassion.
Great Compassion makes a Peaceful Heart.
A Peaceful Heart makes a Peaceful Person.
A Peaceful Person makes a Peaceful Family.
A Peaceful Family makes a Peaceful Community.
A Peaceful Community makes a Peaceful Nation.
A Peaceful Nation makes a Peaceful World.
May all beings live in Happiness and Peace.

—Maha Ghosananda

"You think too much. Too, too much. And then it makes you talk too much. This too much thinking makes spirit sick." These were the words a Buddhist monk spoke to me back in 2011. He was draped in a saffron robe and sitting in the barren yet formal drawing room of an ancient temple in Phnom Penh. I sat before him, and his words caused me to stop sipping my tea. In that moment, I felt like I'd been covered with a warm blanket of compassion and love as he peered straight through my soul. This gracious monk was the first person to accurately see and diagnose my burnout. I shifted my gaze downward to the cool tile floor, thinking that the last time my feet were on cold tiles, I was doing a walk of shame out of the hospital where I'd worked before my surgery. The monk's companion, draped in similar saffron robes, sensed my energy shift, stuffed another bright yellow sweet in his mouth, giggled, and motioned for me to do the same. Heck, if eating this sweet would make me giggle with joy like this monk, give me the platter of these brightly colored Cambodian confections.

The temple where we sat that day had survived the Khmer Rouge, and the monks were disciples of Preah Maha Ghosananda. Ghosananda famously led a 125-mile Dhammayeitra (pilgrimage of truth) across Cambodia in 1992 to begin restoring the hope and spirit of the Cambodian people. The Dhammayeitra continues to this day.

I was divinely guided to take this journey by my breathwork teacher in the United States, Laurie Young. She had graciously invited me at the last minute to join her tour group going to Cambodia, and I jumped at the chance to learn how to meditate and be more mindful. Along with Laurie, I'd join a group of steely-haired and steely-hearted serious yogi women at least 20 years my senior. They were not happy to have a brain doctor join the group. (Back then it seemed that these groups of nosy, and sometimes judgmental, Aunties seemed to follow me everywhere.)

Ironically, my path to meditation started in my postoperative healing period with the cassette tapes given to me by my Aunties. I would listen to the strums of Indian classical music and repeat the Sanskrit chants, even though I had no clue what I was saying. With this chanting, I had noticed an almost immediate improvement in my postoperative chest and abdominal pain, and slowly I was starting to emerge out of the darkness where I'd been lost for so long. Meditation was not something I had been introduced to growing up, let alone learned in my medical training—yet its healing power was profound. Remember, in those days of cassette tapes, there were not yoga studios on every street corner in the United States. Apps were not yet on our phones or smartwatches, reminding us to pause and breathe. Heck, everyone's favorite online university, YouTube, was not populated with gurus reciting their own meditations. To learn more, I had to take my own pilgrimage to my hometown's public library. Yet with all the books I read, I still struggled to find the answers to questions like, how do you get on and stay on the path to inner peace that every spiritual author promises? Hello, could someone please give me the steps one by one? I follow instructions very well (most of the time), but I was doing meditation all wrong, and I couldn't shut down my constant worrying thoughts: *How will I cope with going back to work as a neurologist? Why did I have this achalasia? How do I find love again? Are soulmates even for real?*

Perhaps as I sat in this ancient temple wrapped in that warm blanket of compassion, someone could give me the formula to turn off my constantly analyzing and overachieving Busy Brain. My fervent prayer in traveling all the way to Cambodia was to find the answers.

One of those answers came from the first monk when he said, "No thinking, no talking, just doing." Shifting his saffron robe, he signaled for us to get up and invited us to sit with him and his fellow monks in meditation. I shoved my third confection in my mouth and chewed quickly. We followed the monks and Laurie to the inner temple, where meditation mats lay ready to welcome us. The room was stunning, though to this day I can't remember the specific details of what I saw, only that the marble tiles were cold and there was a silent peace permeating the room unlike any I had ever experienced. A few minutes into the meditation, and your girl here went down for the count. Apparently, I'd flopped from my seated meditation position to a not-so-elegant position flat on the floor, sound asleep and snoring, with saliva from my half-open mouth pooling on the mat. Understandably, Laurie and the oh-so-serious yogi Aunties were angry and mortified, but the giggling monk, who loved to share his sweets, quietly got up, took off the part of his robe that draped his shoulders, and put it on top of me as a blanket. He then patted my arm, looked at Laurie, and said, "She is healing." When Laurie gave me this whole play-by-play later, she told me that in her moment of anger and frustration, she learned one of the most important lessons of her life about compassion—one that could not be taught in any book.

brainSCIENCE Break

The healing sleep I experienced that day in the temple, and on the rest of that trip, changed the way I would think and talk. There were no pagers or phones to wake me up with a patient emergency in the middle of the night. I instead spent my days learning breathwork, practicing meditation, visiting nongovernmental organizations (NGOs) helping women, and sleeping. What I didn't know at the time was that I was on the start of the journey to understand how to face a Busy Brain and cure obsessive, ruminating thinking, anxiety, distraction, and insomnia. I was also starting to get clarity on my questions about stress, burnout, and a Busy Brain. Questions such as, "What is going on physiologically in our Busy Brains when we are on a path to burnout?" and "What do we do to heal burnout when meditation or resilience training is not helping?"

Welcome to section two of *The Busy Brain Cure*. In this section, I not only lay out the symptoms of a Busy Brain (ruminating anxiety, attention deficit disorder, and insomnia) but also dig into the science of why you have these symptoms. In section three, you will get to meet the fearless leaders who admitted they had a Busy Brain and went through the brainSHIFT Protocol to find a path to their healing. Let's not get ahead of ourselves, though. That's a whole other section.

But before we dig in here, first, a word. No, this is not a section about meditation and mindfulness. I know you are here because you need something more than a prescription to another mindfulness class. When people score above a 30 on the Busy Brain Test, one of the first things I hear is how they just can't quiet their Busy Brain to meditate. It's akin to the experience I'd had when I tried to still my mind—though I was exhausted beyond belief, my Busy Brain would not shut down. I was wired and tired, and the voices of the Aunties were haunting me whenever I tried to silence my mind.

A Wired and Tired Busy Brain

What do I mean by being wired and tired? Just that. Basically, you feel "tired," fatigued, or have low energy, and also, at the same time, you are "wired" with nervous or anxious energy.

Here are some of the things I hear from clients who are wired and tired:

1. Don't tell me to meditate. I can't shut down all the racing thoughts, and frankly, I don't want to face those inner demons today.

2. I'm completely exhausted, but at the same time, I have so much nervous energy that I can't sit still, rest, deeply relax, or even sleep soundly.

In clinical terms, being wired and tired means that we are suffering from rumination or worrying that is now interfering with our daily lives.

Rumination in traditional psychological terms is defined as "obsessive thinking about an idea, situation, or choice, especially when it interferes with normal mental functioning." Everyone ruminates, and it is normal when stress levels increase or when you have a deadline coming up.

Rumination that has escalated, however, is ruminating

anxiety—a key symptom of a Busy Brain. With ruminating anxiety, you don't feel calm once the deadline or stressor is over. Ruminating anxiety becomes a problem because it is now frequent, ongoing, or interferes with your ability to engage in daily tasks, concentrate, relate to others, and experience positive emotions. "Why can't I be happy? I do not know what inner peace is. Isn't that just for the woo-woo people who don't have my responsibilities?"

Ruminating anxiety is a pattern that can be distressing and difficult to stop, and usually involves repeating a negative thought or solving an elusive problem. It can look like worrying about a future event, replaying a past scenario, or trying to predict how something will play out. These are the warring conversations happening in your head when you try to sit and breathe or fall asleep.

Ruminating anxiety is controlled by the default mode network (DMN) in the brain. Studies have also found that people with attention deficit hyperactivity disorder (ADHD) have atypical connectivity in the default mode network, which might be associated with distractibility. We will discuss ADHD and ADD later in the book, but ADHD in adults is characterized by symptoms of inattention, impulsivity, and restlessness, resulting in functional impairment. It has been hypothesized that the increased activity in the default mode network may interfere with the function of networks involved in attention and cognitive control. The DMN typically consists of the medial prefrontal cortex (MPFC), posterior cingulate cortex (PCC)/precuneus, inferior parietal lobe (IPL), lateral temporal cortex (LTC), and hippocampal formation (HF). Thus, the default mode network is a group of brain regions that seem to show lower levels of activity when we are engaged in a particular task such as paying attention, and are engaged and working when we're feeling calm, are daydreaming, or are in a place of flow (that ever-elusive inner peace). Furthermore, therapies like meditation have received attention for positively influencing the activity in the default mode network, suggesting this may be part of their mechanism for improving well-being.

So let me summarize: A Busy Brain is a dysfunction of the default mode network, which is a region of multiple areas in the brain. When there is increased activity in one of these areas, it leads to adult-onset attention deficit disorder, ruminating anxiety, and difficulty falling asleep—all the symptoms of a Busy Brain.

We found a similar pattern in our research. Between December 2020 and December 2022, over 16,791 people took the Busy Brain Test online as a part of our research database. A consistent pattern emerged after evaluating these Busy Brain Tests. In addition to sleep difficulties, the consistently highest score emerged in one key area: "I cannot shut down worries, racing thoughts."

What Is Circadian Rhythm, and How Is It Related to a Busy Brain?

Your hypothalamus is the command center that controls the pituitary gland, the autonomic nervous system, and your circadian rhythm. The circadian rhythm is found in the suprachiasmatic nucleus (SCN), a part of the hypothalamus. What is the circadian rhythm? It's the all-important internal clock that controls the cycles in your body, such as sleep, daytime wakefulness, hormones, and body temperature. Every organ system in our body is moderated by circadian rhythms, and they are connected to this master clock.

At different times of the day, the clock genes in the SCN send signals to modulate activity throughout the body. When we are under chronic stress and have neuroinflammation, the circadian rhythm is directly impacted. Your body maintains its biological rhythms through a variety of chemicals at the molecular level in response to your environment. Your light exposure, eating habits, and other environmental cues can maintain or disrupt your biological rhythms. One of the most critical roles our circadian rhythm plays is in our sleep-wake cycle.

Your individual environmental cues are known as zeitgebers, which directly affect the circadian rhythm's internal functioning. The relationship between your physiological and behavioral cues impacts the timing of your sleep-wake cycle. Examples of your personal zeitgebers are the timing of sleep, meals, work, and social interactions.

A distinct pattern of neuroinflammation causes Busy Brain symptoms, and at the core of the problem is a disrupted circadian rhythm. When your circadian rhythm is out of balance, it doesn't only affect your sleep-wake cycle. Once your sleep-wake cycle is off, a secondary disturbance occurs in your core body temperature, cortisol levels, and melatonin secretion.

The circadian rhythm's vast network (or clock cycle) also extends inside and outside your brain. Let's dive deeper into the SCN region. It is a small group of cells lying in the anterior hypothalamus. The electric activity produced in the

SCN has to be transmitted to the rest of the brain and then translated into signals that are received outside the brain by the body's peripheral districts. In subsequent chapters in this section, you will read how the disruption to your circadian rhythm impacts sleep and other organ systems in your body that contribute to a Busy Brain. A disrupted circadian rhythm negatively affects your hormonal health and gut health—specifically stress eating.

The SCN has connections to the pineal gland, which is an important center for the production of melatonin. Your pineal gland releases the highest levels of melatonin when there's darkness and decreases melatonin production when you're exposed to light. In other words, you have low levels of melatonin in your blood during the daylight hours and peak levels of melatonin during the nighttime. The longer the night, the longer your pineal gland secretes melatonin.

Because of this, melatonin has often been referred to as a "sleep hormone." You sleep better when you have the highest levels of melatonin in your body. However, several other factors contribute to your body's ability to sleep and the quality of the sleep you get. Your pineal gland receives information about the daily light-dark (day-night) cycle from the retinas in your eyes and then releases melatonin accordingly. People with blindness who can't detect light usually have irregularly synchronized melatonin cycles leading to circadian rhythm disorders.

Signs That Your Circadian Rhythm Is Out of Balance

Sleep disorders linked to the circadian rhythm are often over-looked and can extend inflammation and imbalances in the rest of your body. Circadian rhythm sleep disorders are typically a misalignment between your sleep timeline and the physical and social 24-hour environmental cycle. This means when you start the habit of setting a regular time to sleep and wake up, the disrupted circadian rhythm will still show up as difficulty falling asleep and staying asleep.

What are common ways we inadvertently send our circadian rhythm out of balance? Whether it is jet lag, working a late shift, or being awake at irregular hours to care for your child, sleep disruption is an inevitable challenge. If these sleep disruptive patterns occur consistently on top of episodic or chronic stress, we are laying down the foundation for a Busy Brain. The first symptoms that may appear are

- Insomnia

- General sleepiness or fatigue

- Indigestion

- Irritability

- Lack of focus.

In addition, our research results showed that the most common symptoms under chronic stress were as follows:

1. Difficulty falling asleep

2. Waking up in the middle of the night, and unable to return to sleep

3. Difficulty focusing and paying attention during the daytime

4. Lack of energy during the daytime

In summary, one of the root causes of having a Busy Brain is disruptions of your circadian rhythm. In the following chapters, we will break down how each root cause of a Busy Brain is rooted in circadian rhythm dysfunction.

Sleep Hygiene to Reset Your Brain's Biological Clock

Is there a way to reset your internal biological rhythm? The foundation of the brainSHIFT 8-week protocol is completing microhabits to reset and restore your circadian rhythm. In addition, we look for health and medical issues that may be contributing to or a cause of the imbalance.

Most individuals with whom I meet at speaking engagements and in the course of corporate wellness consulting have already "tried everything" before joining the 8-week brainSHIFT Program. How about you? One of the quickSHIFTs in section one was an exercise to help you mindfully assess what you have tried in the past and what may or may not have worked for you.

Any treatment protocol for insomnia symptoms ideally should start with visiting your primary care physician (if you haven't already done so) to be screened for a genetic circadian rhythm sleep disorder or obstructive sleep apnea as a cause of your insomnia. Once those have been ruled out, if you have a Busy Brain and want to jump off the stimulant-sedative cycle, the brainSHIFT Protocol was designed for this reason.

In both the traditional medical and integrative medicine spheres, the first step to treating insomnia is not sedative prescription medications. Clinical guidelines published in 2015 in the *Annals of Internal Medicine* recommend cognitive behavioral therapy for insomnia (CBT-I or CBTI) as a first-line treatment.

In chapter 11, I will cover the supplements that have been found to be clinically beneficial for a Busy Brain, including 5-hydroxytryptophan (5-HTP) and magnesium glycinate. I will also discuss the pros and cons of taking melatonin as a supplement, and why long-term use of melatonin can actually disrupt your sleep and circadian rhythm. In chapter 11, we will also start the 7-day sleep challenge, which incorporates CBT-I and the following sleep hygiene recommendations to restore your circadian rhythm.

To keep your biological rhythms in balance, on time, and consistent, the following behaviors are recommended (and yes, I know it can be challenging to find time for these in our professional lives).

- Stand, walk, and be outdoors (if possible) in the sunlight early in your day without sunglasses to reinforce your brain's circadian rhythm's cycle of wakefulness.

- Go to bed and wake up at the same time every day.

- Exercise during the day to make sleeping at night easier and to re-energize your waking hours.

- Avoid caffeine after noon to make sure you can fall asleep.

- Avoid artificial light from electronic devices before bed. We will discuss how we came up with the 30- to 60-minute time frame in subsequent chapters.

- Avoid naps longer than 90 minutes, and don't nap at least 6 hours prior to bedtime.

If our Busy Brains are in overdrive, accomplishing any of the above recommendations may feel overwhelming. You may also have your brain's version of judgmental Aunties snapping back, "Don't you think we are smart and have tried these sleep tips already to no avail?" In section three of this book, I will walk you through the week-by-week process of picking one clear microhabit to do in a manner that will feel like my Aunties invited your brain's Aunties into their living room for an afternoon tea party. The disruption of our brain's circadian rhythm from chronic stress and burnout did not appear overnight. Adopting a mindset of seeking a quick fix will only fuel the cycle of false hope and deep disappointment. In the Busy Brain Cure, you will not find that quick fix, a pill for your ill, or a supplement for all your symptoms. I started to learn this patience and sense of pause to self-reflect during my period of immersion in learning the basics of mindfulness and yoga.

brainPAUSE to Stop the Busy Brain

How many times have we felt so anxious or filled with ruminating thoughts that we cannot focus on controlled breathing exercises or meditation? When rumination and anxiety are heightened in a Busy Brain, it's as if our brains have already jumped off the cliff, so there is no point in saying, "Back up. You don't want to fall off the edge."

Initially, I started offering meditation in week 4 of the brainSHIFT Protocol, and it fell flat. We needed something in addition that targeted Busy Brain. I call it taking a brain-PAUSE. I combine both brain science and mindfulness-based techniques to show you how to engage the default mode network to create a brainPAUSE. In section three, you will learn the specific steps of a brainPAUSE in week 4 of the brainSHIFT Protocol.

I found my path to creating a brainPAUSE after teaching mindfulness programs to large teams and organizations of fellow Busy Brain leaders who would consistently say things like, "What am I doing wrong? I can't shut down my racing thoughts." I felt their pain as those are the same challenges I first experienced, and still sometimes do when I practice meditation.

We weren't doing anything wrong. The brain does not shut down its ability to engage the senses, think, and analyze unless you are under general anesthesia, in a coma, or dead. Taming our Busy Brains teaches us not to react to every last thought, especially those of the judgmental Aunties.

When I needed to silence my brain, I learned to start with reconnecting my brain to my body, i.e., getting out of my own head. Yoga was a path that helped, in addition to running. I remember wanting to learn more about yoga—not just asanas but also pranayama and meditation. In 2012, I found a yoga teacher training program that lasted 8 weeks that would require me to take a prolonged brainPAUSE from work. I was working in a different community hospital job that I had taken after my surgery. I was now stuck filing complex paperwork explaining my leave. In the section "Reason for Leave," I made the mistake of writing "yoga teacher training." It wasn't long after when I was paged to the offices of the chief medical officer, who was stammering to get his words out as he held my request for leave application.

"Is there something you want to tell us? Yoga teacher training? Do you have an alcohol or drug problem, and are going to rehab? Please tell us the truth about why you need 8 weeks off from your clinic and hospital duties. If you are going to rehab, we will support you to avoid losing your medical license."

I couldn't believe it. I was being judged by the toxic medical system just like those steely-haired oh-so-serious yogi Aunties. They were all wondering, why would a brain doctor take yoga teacher training?

I was perplexed and shared the chief medical officer's reaction with my teacher, Gerhard Gessner, a retired engineer from Germany who founded and teaches at Prana Yoga in La Jolla, California. He didn't focus on the "celebrity yoga style" but taught pure hatha yoga honoring the ancestors of India, where yoga originated. He paused, then said, "You think too much. Isn't yoga spiritual rehab?"

During my years of immersing myself learning the basics of mindfulness, meditation, and yoga, I would often see the now popular quote, "When the student is ready, the teacher will appear. When the student is truly ready, the teacher will disappear," that has been attributed to both Buddhist and Tao Te Ching's teachings. While I spent years researching and learning the medical science behind the protocol in this book, I also lived with chronic stress that led to a Busy Brain and burnout. The solution did not just come to me by reading a few medical textbooks and medical journal articles. In this section, in addition to the science of the cure, you are hearing the stories of my teachers, mentors, and guides who played a part in my healing, growing, and learning.

As a professional speaker, I have always heard the adage that "facts tell, but stories sell."

When I would hear that analytical professionals were in my audience—such as fellow physicians, engineers, or computer science professionals—I would add an extra eleven slides of data and cut the stories and anecdotes almost completely out of my talk. I would see bored faces or the faces of individuals frantically taking notes and feeling stressed in keeping up with the science. And if a meeting event professional told me to cut out all the science talk to keep the energy light, fun, and motivational...the session would feel like fluff.

Over time, I learned that my style has been to avoid the fluff and overstuff my presentations with a healthy mix of both stories and data. As you start the journey with me in this scientific section of the book, I hope that bringing together both the stories and the science will help you feel motivated to start and continue the 8-week brainSHIFT Protocol in section three of the book. For those of you who have a Busy Brain and want to jump ahead to section three of the book, the reasoning and the order may not make sense without understanding the logic, facts, and research behind each action. I continue to share the stories of my healing journey not only so that you may see yourself in my actions and behaviors, but also to honor the teachers and guides who showed up on my path to restore health.

Once I learned to brainSHIFT my own Busy Brain and helped thousands of clients do the same, I came to one conclusion that shapes my life as a leader. To live life well, we are simultaneously the teacher and the student of life.

brainDUMP Chapter 5 Summary

1. Are you feeling both wired and tired? A Busy Brain can make you feel exhausted while simultaneously feeling like you cannot stop your never-ending to-do lists from playing on a loop in your brain.

2. Ruminating anxiety is a hallmark symptom of a Busy Brain. Ruminating anxiety means you still have obsessive and intrusive thoughts when a stressful event or deadline is over.

3. A disruption of your brain's circadian rhythm is the root cause of a Busy Brain.

4. Sleep hygiene is the foundation of resetting your brain's circadian rhythm.

5. A brainPAUSE is an exercise that combines both mindfulness-based stress reduction techniques and

THE BUSY BRAIN CURE

brain science. Taking a brainPAUSE can help you shut down all the racing thoughts (ruminating anxiety) during the day so you can find focus.

6

Hormones in a Busy Brain

One day during my yoga teacher training, I plopped down in savasana on my mat in the back of the studio. I'd taken up residence daily in a spot right under the window that offered me a peek of the perfectly manicured palm-tree-lined street of La Jolla. But on this day, something else interrupted that familiar position...a voice. One I did not recognize. I was used to the typical voices of my judgmental, funny, and wise Aunties, but this voice was different. It told me bluntly and clearly to quit my traditional neurology job. I questioned my sanity, thinking that the rigorous 8 hours of yoga, meditation, and studying in yoga teacher training were doing something to my brain, but that didn't feel quite right. I mean, it was doing something to my brain, but not in a bad way. Gerhard had been right. Yoga *is* spiritual rehab.

I was now physically removed from my routine schedule in a busy world of practicing physician and dutiful daughter to one of prolonged silences. I hadn't had access to Google searches, well-meaning family members, or bosses at work ordering me around the whole time I'd been in the training. I was also avoiding social media, online news, and television. With distracting external voices removed from my life, I started to connect with my own thoughts, process my emotions, and then enjoy the silence. The silence is where the voice started, the one that told me to quit my traditional neurology job.

I was simply learning to be still in my brain and body, and by doing so, now I was hearing the voice of intuition and wisdom, what I called my inner soul compass. And of course, your girl argued back. *What do you mean, quit my job? I am not going to quit medicine to teach yoga. If I did, I couldn't afford these Lululemon cropped leggings with the matching tank top.*

But later that night, back in my room, another chunk of my hair fell out; the hair loss and acne had been progressing since I got sick and went through surgery. If this wasn't evidence that something needed to change, I didn't know what was. My inner soul compass whispered what I'd already known deep down for over a decade—something was wrong with my thyroid gland. In the past, I'd read the symptoms of underperforming or low thyroid hormones, and I checked almost every box. I'd even discussed it with my primary care doctor, who said, "your TSH (thyroid-stimulating hormone) is within the normal range. Hair loss is normal; you are probably just stressed." However, I couldn't help but feel that there was nothing normal about the roller-coaster ride my hormones and I were on together. Now I was sure.

When I returned home from yoga teacher training, I had gained a fresh perspective and a calmer demeanor, but I did not quit my job. Not just yet. However, I did listen to my inner soul compass and found a new primary care doctor, hoping he would listen to me when I told him something was wrong with my hormones even if my TSH levels were in the normal range. I decided before my visit that I would demand, as a doctor and patient, that he draw additional thyroid labs, even if insurance wouldn't pay for them.

To my gratitude, I did not have to demand anything. This kind elderly gentleman listened to me and my inner soul compass without judgment. Not only had he known of my work as a neurologist in the community, but his nurse had attended one of my yoga and breathing classes in the hospital and enjoyed it, so he knew of my desire to bring my learnings from meditation, mindfulness, and yoga into healthcare. He shared with me that he had started a journey of taking classes for physicians at the University of Arizona Andrew Weil Center for Integrative Medicine. He then listened to my long history of gastrointestinal issues, surgery for achalasia, and decade-long battle to convince someone that my thyroid was off.

Unfortunately, not only were my inner soul compass and I right, but the news was even more troubling. In addition to abnormal levels of several of my thyroid labs, I also had a dangerously low vitamin D3 level (below 20) that he attributed to my chronic use of antacid medications before I'd had my surgery. At that time in traditional medicine, a healthy level was considered above 30. We both agreed that I needed to find an expert to help with my hormones, but in the meantime, I read a lot of scientific articles about the super vitamin D3 and how it affected not only bones, but brain and hormones.

In my search for a hormone expert, I realized I wanted to find someone who was not only up to date on the science of hormonal health, but who could also teach me to be a better doctor for my patients in regard to their hormones. The more I dug into my search for the right doctor, the more I found out about the role hormones play in our mood, ability to pay attention, and sleep. (I'll share more of that later.)

I finally found my doctor in the most unlikely place imaginable. There he was, without a shirt on, leaning against a motorcycle, in an ad in an in-flight magazine. Dr. Jeffry Life. He was clearly targeting male executives in search of their libido and pre-midlife crisis bodies while they chugged Woodford Reserve during their Busy-Brained business class flights. Dr. Jeffry Life was the chief medical officer of a company called Cenegenics. Cenegenics is one of the first health and wellness companies in precision and preventative medicine. In the fine print of the ad, however, there was something about how Cenegenics also treated women's hormones. I showed the magazine ad to one of my Aunties who had been following my journey into holistic health and integrative medicine. I was later summoned for a cup of chai in her formal living room, and then the inquisition started. "You want to go to this 72-year-old Babaji (old man) with abdomens like a 26-year-old bodybuilder? Ho hai, this must be Photograph-shopped. You are a brain doctor...do you see a helmet? No. Hai, why would you go there? His treatment will make you grow a beard, and you will never find a suitable husband." Once again, the judgmental Auntie was a mirror for the fear I had in my own brain to try something new and different, something off the beaten path to what I had been taught in traditional medical school and residency training.

Thankfully I followed my inner soul compass to reach out to the company. It turns out that not only did Cenegenics take female patients, but they were also training doctors of all specialties on hormonal health to promote health and longevity—the two things I'd been looking for in my search. And I could keep my blouse on.

brainSCIENCE Break

You've reached this chapter because you have likely already tried a meditation app, supplements your bestie swore by, and a random cleanse you only finished halfway before you got tired of staring at the tiles on your bathroom floor. And nothing has helped so far. Maybe your own inner soul compass is telling you that something is off just as mine did. I hear from so many who scored above a 30 on the Busy Brain Test tell me, "Dr. Romie, my sleep is fine, but I still feel like someone robs me of my energy during the day." Maybe you fall asleep and stay asleep (for the most part), but you still have difficulty focusing or you feel anxiety during the day. I hear you. I see you. And I believe you. Something may still be off balance.

(Note: if you missed the invitation to take the free Busy Brain Test in section one of this book, you can take a brainPAUSE here and go to *www.BusyBrainCure.com* and take the test for free. A score above 30 indicates that you may have a Busy Brain.)

In the last chapter, we addressed a disturbed circadian

rhythm as one of the root causes of a Busy Brain. When your circadian rhythm is out of balance, it doesn't only affect your sleep-wake cycle. The circadian rhythm's vast network extends inside and outside of your brain. I discussed the SCN—the suprachiasmatic nucleus—which is a small group of cells lying in the anterior hypothalamus. The electric activity produced in the SCN has to be transmitted to the rest of the brain and then be translated into signals that are received outside the brain by the peripheral districts of the body. The SCN communicates signals in three ways:

1. Neuronal networking, by directly making contact with several other brain regions.

2. Chemically, by synthesizing signaling molecules.

3. Indirectly, by setting rest-activity rhythms that in turn trigger feeding-fasting cycles.

When any of the messaging systems of the SCN fail to function, it negatively impacts your hormonal health. Hormones are not only in your sex organs (testosterone, estrogen, progesterone) but also in your brain, thyroid, and adrenal glands. There are over fifty other hormones in your body that regulate all your organs' functioning.

Several hormones are known to be dependent on or function through daily signaling from the SCN. Examples of the most studied of these hormones are melatonin, cortisol, gonadal steroids, prolactin, thyroid hormone, and growth hormone. We discussed the important role of melatonin controlling your sleep-wake cycle in the previous chapter. While all these hormones affect your brain and physical health, when it comes to symptoms of a Busy Brain, thyroid hormone balance is crucial.

There are several other nutrient-sensitive hormones that also depend on your circadian rhythm, namely insulin, leptin, ghrelin, and adiponectin. All of these hormones govern your hunger and metabolism, and we will discuss them in the next chapter when we discuss how to biohack your nutrition.

We'll set many of those hormones aside in this chapter and focus on the role of your thyroid hormones in a Busy Brain. In addition, I will also cover vitamin D3 as a star player in this book. I am one of many colleagues in the integrative medicine community who say that vitamin D3 did not get its full credit when named, and in addition to a critical vitamin is a super prohormone, meaning that it promotes healthy levels of hormones.

Before you go googling how to take an online test for symptoms concerning a potential thyroid or vitamin D3 imbalance, I am here to tell you as a physician that the only way to truly ascertain if you have an issue is to have your labs drawn. Again, I know a Busy Brain can tempt us for a quick fix like ordering a supplement online and calling it a day. I want you to find the root cause of your Busy Brain, and to have an accurate picture, partner with a trusted healthcare provider and ask for these lab evaluations. Having recent lab results in regard to your vitamin D3 levels and a full thyroid panel can help us create an accurate picture of the hormones and chemistries in your body.

Star of the brainSHIFT: Vitamin D3

Vitamin D (also referred to as "calciferol") is a fat-soluble vitamin that is naturally present in a few foods, added to others, and available as a dietary supplement. Vitamin D has several forms. Vitamin D2 and D3 are the most important of these. Vitamin D is also produced endogenously (in our bodies) through our exposure to natural sunlight. When ultraviolet (UV) rays from sunlight strike the skin, it triggers a process of multiple steps through the body for conversion of precursors of vitamin D to transform into vitamin D3 (also known as cholecalciferol). Vitamin D2 has a slightly different molecular structure and is derived from plants, whereas vitamin D3 is derived from animal sources. In clinical studies, vitamin D3 is shown to be more clinically effective when taken as a supplement compared to vitamin D2. In this chapter, when I refer to vitamin D, I am discussing vitamin D3 unless otherwise discussed.

I will say that vitamin D3 has been mislabeled and undersold on its value to human health. When something has the name "vitamin," we often miss the importance of its role in modulating every hormone interaction in our brain and body. Vitamin D3 has traditionally been known to help the body absorb and retain calcium and phosphorus, which are both critical for bone structure and health. Also, studies show that vitamin D3 can reduce cancer cell growth, help control infections, and reduce inflammation, including in the brain, known as neuroinflammation. Its deficiency has been linked to many brain and mental health diseases, such as dementia, depression, diabetes mellitus, autism, and schizophrenia.

People with deficient vitamin D3 levels are at increased risk for multiple sclerosis relapses, multiple types of cancer, and cognitive decline. These were known facts that I was taught in my neurology residency training even in the late 1990s.

But let's talk about how we as humans get all forms of vitamin D, metabolize it, and measure it correctly.

Sunshine and Vitamin D

UV-B rays from the sun are the best direct source of vitamin D for your health. Unfortunately, due to lack of sun exposure or use of sunblock, up to 90% of Americans are estimated to have low levels of vitamin D3 in their blood. So, how much sun exposure do you need? If you have fair skin, it is estimated that you need at least 10 minutes of sun exposure daily without using sunblock or protective clothing on all four limbs of your body. It is said that an estimate of 10 minutes of exposure equals 10,000 IU (international units). If you have darker skin, the melanin in your skin slows down the production of vitamin D with sun exposure, and it is recommended that you spend at least 40 minutes in the sunshine daily without sunscreen. Now, I will say this: neither I nor any of my dermatology colleagues would recommend this much skin exposure without protection from UV rays due to increased risk of skin cancer. Therefore, it is important to find another source of vitamin D3.

Food Sources of Vitamin D

Vitamin D can also be derived from food, but it cannot reach the level of vitamin D that sun exposure provides.

Foods rich in vitamin D include:

- Halibut

- Carp

- Mackerel

- Eel

- Salmon

- Whitefish

- Swordfish

- Rainbow trout

- Cod liver oil

- Sardines

- Tuna

- Portobello mushrooms (exposed to UV light)

- Maitake mushrooms (exposed to UV light)

- Eggs

- Raw milk

Vitamin D Deficiency and Your Busy Brain

There is a researched link between vitamin D deficiency and the symptoms of a Busy Brain: anxiety, ADHD, and insomnia.

Vitamin D and Anxiety

Multiple studies have found that vitamin D deficiency may increase anxiety. One study gave participants with vitamin D deficiency supplements for 6 months while another group didn't receive any supplements. They used a test called the Hamilton Anxiety Rating Scale-14 to measure participants' level of anxiety. Ultimately, vitamin D3 supplements significantly helped lessen symptoms of anxiety in the group that received them as opposed to the group that didn't take any vitamin D3 supplementation at all.

The *Journal of Diabetes Research* conducted a study to see if supplements could improve mental health and type 2 diabetes. Forty-six women participated in the study for 6 months and completed a survey about their mental health. The study found that taking vitamin D3 supplements significantly decreased anxiety levels in women suffering from type 2 diabetes.

Yet another study found that those suffering from anxiety had lower levels of calcidiol, which is the precursor of vitamin D3. Broken down, vitamin D produces the by-product calcidiol. The study notes that low vitamin D levels are thought to increase the chances of depression, diabetes, and cancer. The study also notes that literature from thousands of years ago hints at the link between vitamin D deficiency and anxiety.

Vitamin D and ADHD

In a meta-analysis of research studies of children with ADHD, it was consistently found that children with ADHD had lower vitamin D3 levels compared to those without the diagnosis. Moreover, lower perinatal and childhood vitamin D status were both associated with a higher likelihood of developing ADHD. This means if a child's vitamin D levels were low at birth or early childhood, there was a higher risk of developing ADHD. Now, I am not saying that children should stop taking prescribed medications from their doctors for ADHD. I am simply stating there is also an important role of vitamin D that has been shown in maintaining cognitive functions of attention.

In adults, there are now over two decades of research showing a cognitive decline associated with a low vitamin D level, but what about the ability to pay attention or adult-onset attention deficit disorder (ADD)? We lack the studies at this time to show the specific correlation of vitamin D3 supplementation with adult-onset ADD, but we can only extrapolate from the numerous studies done with children.

Vitamin D and Insomnia

Vitamin D deficiency is associated with sleep disorders and poor sleep quality. Through a meta-analysis of observational studies involving 9,397 participants, Qui Gao and his research team found that participants with vitamin D deficiency had an increased likelihood of sleep disorders, poor sleep quality, and shorter sleep duration. They also provided evidence that serum vitamin D levels (measured by checking 25-hydroxyvitamin D levels) below 20 ng/mL could significantly heighten the odds of unhealthy sleep. Multiple other extensive studies have yielded similar results that low vitamin D levels affect the quantity and quality of sleep. In a large review article, it has been shown that there is efficacy in supplementing vitamin D3 to improve sleep, but there is inadequate research to show benefits of supplementation with vitamin D2.

Lab Evaluation for Vitamin D Deficiency

Laboratory testing to assess your vitamin D levels consists of fasting blood tests. These labs can be ordered by your primary care physician and are traditionally covered by your health insurance.

- 1,25-dihydroxyvitamin D

- 25-hydroxyvitamin D

Additional labs that may get tested in relation to symptoms of vitamin D deficiency:

- Liver function tests

- hs-CRP (highly sensitive C-reactive protein)

- Parathyroid hormone tests

- Serum calcium levels

What Is the Correct Vitamin D Level in Adults?

Controversy remains between the traditional medical community and the progressive integrative/functional medicine community about your vitamin D levels. In addition, there is controversy about the FDA's guideline of needing only 400 to 800 IU of vitamin D daily.

There has not been an exact number or range of serum concentrations that are linked to a specific disease—for example, if your 25-hydroxyvitamin D levels are X, you will have rickets or a bone fracture in your hip. An expert committee from the Food and Nutrition Board (FNB) at the National Academies of Sciences, Engineering, and Medicine (NASEM) did provide conclusions based on the medical evidence that summarized the following:

1. If your 25-hydroxyvitamin D levels are below 30 nmol/L (less than 12 ng/mL), you have vitamin D deficiency.

2. Some people are potentially at risk of bone disease when their 25-hydroxyvitamin D levels fall between 30 and 50 nmol/L (12 to 20 ng/mL). This level is known as vitamin D inadequacy.

3. If your 25-hydroxyvitamin D is 50 nmol/L (20 ng/mL) or higher, you have what is considered sufficient Vitamin D levels.

4. The Endocrine Society recommends a different number, saying that a serum 25-hydroxyvitamin D needs to be at least 75 nmol/L (30 ng/mL) for adequate bone health.

A general rule I was taught in neurology is to treat the person's symptoms and not their labs. This means it is important to not make an assumption on lab numbers alone, unless they are at an extreme level compared to the normal range. Instead, it is important to talk to a person and learn about their symptoms and complete a physical examination. Numbers alone don't tell the complete story.

To Cure a Busy Brain, we follow the medical literature for men and women that shows optimized cognitive and mood function—that is, a powerful memory and sense of calm—which is a level between 80-100 nmol/L.

Vitamin D Supplementation

Vitamin D supplements are available as vitamin D2 (D2) and vitamin D3 (D3). Both versions can be used to treat vitamin D deficiency, but D3 is consistently more effective than D2 in research studies, especially regarding brain and mental health symptoms. This is likely because in pharmacological studies in humans, D3 increased total and free 25-hydroxyvitamin D levels to a greater extent than D2. How much vitamin D3 should you take? We make additional recommendations based on your lab values inside the brainSHIFT 8-week course; however, please discuss your labs and the correct dose of daily vitamin D3 with your physician. In the brainSHIFT Protocol, when a 25-hydroxyvitamin D level is low or borderline low, we typically dose vitamin D3 at 5,000 to 10,000 IU daily.

Thyroid Hormone Disorder

For both men and women, the thyroid gland is a key component of all our metabolic functions for the brain and the body. In particular for the Busy Brain Cure, we focus on the role of the thyroid gland in maintaining the function of mood, energy, and attention.

Thyroid hormone levels can be low (hypothyroidism) or high (hyperthyroidism). Both hypothyroidism and hyperthyroidism are root causes of Busy Brain. We also know when the circadian rhythm is off, one of the important hormonal pathways affected is that of our thyroid gland.

How Common Is Thyroid Disease?

In the latest epidemiology studies in the US, the prevalence of overt hypothyroidism varies from 0.1 to 2% of adults. The prevalence of subclinical hypothyroidism is higher, ranging from 4 to 10% of adults, with possibly a higher frequency in older women. In fact, hypothyroidism is five to eight times more common in women than men, and more common in women with small body sizes at birth and during childhood.

Traditional hypothyroid symptoms (low thyroid hormone levels) are associated with weight gain and constipation. (Hair loss is also common and too often dismissed by traditional medicine as a vanity complaint.) But hypothyroidism symptoms can also include anxiety. In fact, a review published in June 2018 in *JAMA Psychiatry* (*Journal of the American Medical Association*) found that people with hypothyroidism are more than twice as likely as people without the condition to develop anxiety disorders and that 29.8% of all anxiety disorders are associated with autoimmune thyroid disease.

Hyperthyroidism was found in 1.2% (0.5% overt and 0.7% subclinical) of patients. Hyperthyroid symptoms are nonspecific and may be present in patients with the subclinical disease and absent in those with an overt disease, especially older adults. Most patients with overt hyperthyroidism have obvious symptoms that include anxiety, emotional lability, weakness, tremor, palpitations, heat intolerance, increased perspiration, and weight loss despite a normal or increased appetite.

I want to highlight a point on which all the medical literature agrees (both traditional endocrinologists and integrative medicine doctors): thyroid disease is underdiagnosed. Could this be you or someone else you know with a Busy Brain? It is estimated that one in eight people have thyroid disease that is getting missed because their symptoms are not obvious. Or they are like me and their TSH levels are in the normal range, despite symptoms of thyroid issues.

Thyroid disease can promote the occurrence of other symptoms of a Busy Brain, including insomnia and ADD/ADHD. Research shows that those with generalized resistance to thyroid hormones are far more likely to have ADHD when compared to other family members with healthy thyroid functions. Another large meta-analysis assessed that hyperthyroidism and hypothyroidism have clinical overlap with sleep conditions such as insomnia, restless legs syndrome, and obstructive sleep apnea. In other words, well-established symptoms of nervousness, anxiety, and insomnia are related to both hyperthyroidism and subclinical hypothyroidism.

THE BUSY BRAIN CURE

Too often, a thyroid disorder is missed by a physician because of vague symptoms given by the patient, and only one laboratory value is checked—the thyroid-stimulating hormone (TSH). As a part of a routine screening, a doctor will see that your TSH is within a broad normal range from 0.4 to 4.0 mIU/L. Without a more comprehensive lab evaluation for your thyroid gland, it cannot be said that "your thyroid function is normal." Too often, key symptoms—such as lack of daytime energy, and anxiety—are dismissed as "stress" without digging deeper to assess if the thyroid gland is the culprit.

In our lab panel for the brainSHIFT Protocol, I recommend that you ask your physician to order a full thyroid panel that includes the following laboratory values:

1. Thyroid-stimulating hormone (TSH)

2. Total triiodothyronine T3

3. Total thyroxine T4

4. Free triiodothyronine (fT3)

5. Free thyroxine (fT4)

6. Reverse T3 (rT3)

7. Anti-thyroglobulin antibodies

8. Thyroid peroxidase antibodies

When we run this 8-week brainSHIFT program for corporate teams, inevitably some participants return and say their physician was not sure all of these labs were needed. I often email or call their physicians to explain why this thorough

screening is needed. Without that entire lab panel, the following root causes of a Busy Brain can be missed:

1. Autoimmune thyroiditis

2. Subclinical hypothyroidism

3. Subclinical hyperthyroidism

So why aren't more people, including myself back in the
day, getting their full thyroid panels screened by their physicians? In my clinical days, a thyroid disorder had to show
physical symptoms, such as weight gain and constipation,
for a doctor to consider treatment. A primary care doctor or
endocrinologist did not consider neurological and psychiatric
symptoms of ADHD, anxiety, and insomnia as part of a thyroid disorder. Suppose these are the primary symptoms you
have and you do not have the physical symptoms of thyroid
imbalance. In that case, clinical studies show a primary care
doctor is less likely to treat your thyroid disease. Instead, you'll
hear what I did all those years ago: "You are just a stressed-
out type A personality…" Sure, and by the way, when I got
my full evaluation with the Cenegenics hormone doctors, to
no one's surprise, I had autoimmune Hashimoto's thyroiditis.
Autoimmune thyroid disease can often present with a TSH
in a normal range while your immune system is attacking
your thyroid gland like it is a foreign invader. The doctors at
the Cenegenics clinic started me on medication at age thirty-
seven, and for the first time in my life, I had energy and regular periods. I try not to go back and play the if-only game,
wondering what would have happened if this was caught in

my twenties when I was in medical school. Would I have been less stressed? Would I have ended up with such severe achalasia? Would I have been able to get pregnant?

How different would my life be? The what-if or if-only game is dangerous and made even worse when we have a Busy Brain. Now I consider that I had to journey through my mess in order to help you clean up yours.

The voice of my internal soul compass eventually became so loud, even when I was back in my day-to-day hectic life, that I would openly say I'd be leaving clinical medicine when my contract came up for renewal. And I did. When my journey to connect Western medicine and Eastern traditions became clearer, I left my traditional neurology job in 2013. This time, however, there was no walk of shame like when I left my academic clinical neurology job. I saw a path in front of me that would require me to start my own business and figure out a way to bring root cause medicine (integrative medicine) to brain and mental health disease patients.

I went and studied integrative medicine and took my board exams. It was glorious to walk into a room full of colleagues at the American Board of Integrative and Holistic Medicine (ABIHM, now known as AIHM) who didn't judge me for meditating, doing yoga, and optimizing my nutrition. Instead, I felt a sense of welcome and common purpose.

When I began my new career as an integrative medicine physician and entrepreneur, I knew I would need to prioritize my health above all else. My journey to keep my hormones healthy continued when I moved to Orlando, Florida, and went under the care of one of my partners, Dr. Thomas

Moracewskei, in the integrative medicine clinic where I'd started to see clients. He was another compassionate physician with an ob-gyn background who then did years of additional training in hormonal health. He was a renowned faculty member of the American Academy of Anti-Aging Medicine and was known as the Jedi Master of Hormones. His healing and wisdom went far, but I most remember him for simply saying, "You cannot heal the stress and pain of others without first healing the negative impact of stress on your own hormones and immune system." I honor him today as he bravely lost his battle with prostate cancer in 2020. I would not be healthy and believe so deeply in my mission if it wasn't for him.

Thanks to him, my biggest brainSHIFT has been to take care of my brain and body first. Then I can take care of business in my unapologetic, type A, success-driven way. Thank you, Jedi Master.

brainDUMP Chapter 6 Summary

- A key foundational abnormality in a Busy Brain is a disrupted circadian rhythm.

- Circadian rhythm is responsible for not only your sleep-wake cycle but also the cycle and feedback loop of all of your hormones.

- A key hormone imbalance in a Busy Brain is thyroid disease.

- Both hyperthyroid and hypothyroid disease can lead

to symptoms of a Busy Brain, and both are underdiagnosed because often neurological and mental health symptoms are dismissed.

• None of your hormones (nor many of your cognitive focusing skills) can be optimized without a healthy vitamin D level.

7

Inflammation, Sugar, and Caffeine in a Busy Brain

"Do you have a special family recipe for angel food cake?" Dr. Paul Pritchard III asked his epilepsy patient, who was tucked into his hospital bed with his wife seated by his side. They both hesitated, wondering why Dr. Pritchard (the head neurologist on call) would ask such a thing early in the morning. And then they smiled, and a deep conversation ensued as to whether vanilla extract or almond extract was the key. They all reminded me of my Aunties sitting over a cup of chai debating recipes—Ginger? Cardamom? You put a cinnamon stick in your chicken biryani? Except here in this hospital room in South Carolina, we'd have to substitute sweet tea for chai.

I looked at the clock on the wall. I had been awake 28.5 hours and counting, standing (or running) around the hospital as the on-call resident physician for neurology. We were now starting attending rounds, which meant Dr. Pritchard had not only me but two other resident physicians, an intern, two medical students, the nurse, and the case manager cramped in this hospital room, trying to focus and appear to be taking notes on the recipe exchange. We were one dog short of a Southern family reunion.

"Oh, y'all are from Hampton? Well, I have a third cousin by marriage in Hampton..." Dr. Pritchard said, switching the conversation from angel food to ancestors.

My legs were about to give out, and my frizzy, curly hair smelled like Chick-fil-A french fries (my post-call breakfast in the hospital cafeteria). I didn't know if fried potatoes would give me sustenance, but I needed to get through conversations like this for the remaining thirteen patients on the unit. I looked at my carefully organized notes about every neurology patient we were about to visit. I knew their diagnosis, labs, brain scan results, overnight vitals, and whether they peed, pooped, or vomited, but I had neglected the "angel food cake factor."

When rounding, Dr. Pritchard had this intuitive way of seeking out a secret family recipe, gossip about long-lost family members, or shared ancestors in South Carolina. The "angel food cake factor" was his way of disarming a patient with genuine compassion and hospitality, so he could assess neurological and mental status. He is a brilliant doctor, and when he found a common ground, typically around food, patients and their family members would start to feel comfortable in what is an overwhelming process of being admitted to the hospital and being treated for a brain, spine, or psychiatric disease. And to no one's surprise, once patients were made comfortable, he could then ask them about the details of their often complicated medical history to help make a complete diagnosis. He was always able to quickly ascertain important clinical details that we had missed overnight, no matter how long we spent trying to talk to the patients ourselves.

Don't let his talk of shared family ancestry or where the best barbecue was to be found fool you. Dr. Pritchard was a neurology professor and researcher known around the world for his commitment, leadership, and research in the field of epilepsy. We knew to work on his rotation in our residency training was an honor and one where the hard and long hours would pay off.

When I'd been adopted into the fold by my neurology colleagues at the Medical University of South Carolina with their Southern hospitality, I quickly learned the term "comfort food." In brainSHIFT, we not only recommend comfort food, but we celebrate it. And the Deep South isn't the only place with ties to comfort food either. Anyone on the planet with a joyful memory or positive experience tied to food involving family, ancestry, religious holidays, country, or region of origin knows what comfort food is.

What about my Chick-fil-A french fries for breakfast? Are they comfort food? They can be, but when you add in the fact that I was rewarding myself with them for surviving a stressful night on call in the hospital and I'd been awake for over 24 hours (and doing this every third or fourth night), suffice it to say that my circadian rhythm had lost all sense of night and day. My french fry gobbling in this case was stress eating, and it was all about high glycemic carbohydrates, saturated fats, and salt.

brainSCIENCE Break

Stress eating, also called emotional eating, typically refers to overeating due to feelings of stress or negative emotions. We crave sugary foods, foods high in fat, or salty foods due to changes in the blood sugar and salt levels during chronic stress. In the previous chapters, we discussed how chronic stress leads to neuroinflammation. With neuroinflammation, there is an activation of the hypothalamic–pituitary–adrenal axis (HPA axis).

When the HPA axis is dysregulated in chronic stress, the adrenal gland will keep pumping out a stress hormone known as cortisol. In reaction to this, insulin levels surge in the bloodstream and thus will lower blood sugar levels. So, we end up craving a sugary food that will rapidly increase blood sugar levels. Similarly, those who crave salty foods in the face of chronic stress have also altered sodium, magnesium, and potassium levels due to the adrenal gland pumping out a hormone known as aldosterone. Aldosterone levels rising in the face of stress can trigger the kidneys to dump out critical minerals like sodium and magnesium into the urine instead of preserving it for our optimal hydration.

So yes, as you can see, there is a biochemical and hormonal reason as to why you crave certain foods under chronic stress. The goal is that once we cure your Busy Brain, the neuroinflammation effects of chronic stress will dampen, and your food cravings will lessen and eventually disappear.

Neuroinflammation in a Busy Brain

Inflammation in the brain is known as neuroinflammation. Chronic stress creates neuroinflammation in many pathways in the brain. At the time of chronic stress, the amygdala stimulates the hypothalamus. With the stimulation of the hypothalamus, there is a disruption in the hypothalamic-pituitary–adrenal axis and autonomic dysfunction.

In addition, neuroinflammation disrupts the circadian rhythm, which is one of the root causes of a Busy Brain. Once this happens, neuroinflammation also will trigger inflammatory responses in the body that will wreak havoc in various organ systems, including the pancreas and the rest of the digestive tract. We introduced the topic of neuroinflammation in general in chapter 2; here, I want to specifically discuss how neuroinflammation starts during periods of stress and how a specific pattern of inflammation in your brain causes a Busy Brain.

Let's break down the neurochemistry of neuroinflammation with acute episodic and chronic stress. Scientists have uncovered that with chronic stress, there is an activation of the resident immune cells in the brain known as microglia. These are stimulated to produce inflammatory cytokines, and these particular cytokines (such as interleukin-1, IL-1) are more dangerous in fueling neuroinflammation. Cytokines are signaling proteins that help control inflammation in your body by helping your immune system mount a defense if germs or other substances that can make you sick enter your body. However, too many cytokines can lead to excess inflammation and conditions like autoimmune diseases.

IL-1 is a master regulator of immune cell recruitment and activity in the brain, and this path of neuroinflammation mediates psychopathology, such as mood issues. Basically, the more emotionally stressed we are feeling, there will be a related rise in IL-1 levels, thus fanning the flames of neuroinflammation. This particular pattern of IL-1-mediated inflammation in the brain is seen in relation to anxiety, depression, and feeling burned out. In addition to neuroinflammation raising IL-1 levels, other research shows that critical markers of inflammation that primarily affect the hippocampus and prefrontal cortex of the brain rise during periods of stress. These are the areas that when disrupted lead to difficulty focusing and anxiety.

The elevated pro-inflammatory cytokines in the brain trigger a cascade of negative effects. One of them is the ongoing disruption of the hypothalamic-pituitary-adrenal axis. When the HPA axis is stimulated, it disrupts both hormone systems in the body as well as the autonomic nervous system regulating digestion and hunger.

Important hormones that govern your sense of hunger, fullness, and metabolism are mediated by your circadian rhythm (in the hypothalamus). In chapter 5, we discussed the role of sleep disturbance with circadian rhythm abnormalities, but nutrient-sensitive hormones are also affected. Hormones such as leptin and insulin are dysregulated, and this helps to explain why hunger levels are affected by chronic stress and a Busy Brain.

How do we assess or diagnose neuroinflammation without having to biopsy your brain? A doctor starts by taking a complete history of how you are feeling, and what led you to this

point. Any of my colleagues will tell you, it takes more than the
average 7 minutes a primary care doctor has allotted to spend
with you. (The short office visits are not our fault as doctors,
but a symptom of a broken healthcare system—diving into this
problem will elevate all of our stress levels now.) A thorough
mental health screening and physical examination is also required. In addition to a complete history and physical exam,
to understand neuroinflammation and the root cause of a Busy
Brain, there are specific laboratory tests that must be assessed.
A key laboratory evaluation we use to assess neuroinflammation in a Busy Brain is measuring how your body reacts to stress
by measuring insulin levels, hemoglobin A1c levels, and blood
glucose levels. By assessing these lab values, we look to see if
you have a disease like type 1 or type 2 diabetes mellitus. We
can also assess inflammation in your body and then indirectly
assess how stress is affecting your brain.

State of Your Brain and Blood Sugar

How do you feel after you eat a large piece of a sugary birthday cake or other foods or drinks that have a high amount of
sugar in them? Do you feel a quick energy burst followed by
a crash? This is the effect of blood sugar. It gives you a quick
surge of energy, but what many people aren't aware of is that
high blood sugar is very dangerous for the brain. When a
spike in blood sugar is detected (when we eat said foods), the
autonomic nervous system and pancreas react by pumping
out insulin to get that sugar converted to energy. Over time,
some people can become insulin-resistant, where this mech-

anism no longer works, and they end up with high blood sugar. Traditionally this is known as prediabetes or diabetes.

The regulation of insulin is crucial not only for the pancreas to control your blood sugar but also for the brain. Foods that spike your blood sugar are known as high glycemic foods. High glycemic foods are defined as carbohydrates that are always quickly digested and absorbed, causing a rapid rise in blood sugar. Examples of high glycemic foods are white sugar, white flour, white rice, white potatoes, and white bread. You can see a full list of high glycemic foods in the free resources at *www.BusyBrainCure.com.*

The body breaks down high glycemic foods into two components, glucose and fructose. This is particularly relevant because a part of your brain cells' structures (both neurons and glia) have glucose receptors that are constantly working and the brain's primary energy source. This means that brain cells have genes that are always turned on so that receptors are ready to respond to high sugar levels in the brain. Studies have been conducted on the effects of high sugar levels on the brain. For instance, they blunt your long-term verbal retrieval and facilitation of cognitive executive performance, key components of your focus during intellectual activities that utilize your language and memory skills.

High glycemic foods (I use the term *sugar* interchangeably here) can have a negative impact on your mental health and wellness, particularly when it comes to your ability to maintain a healthy mood and focus.

One of the primary causes of depression is the hormone serotonin (or, more specifically, the lack thereof). Sugar interferes with the brain's and body's ability to produce serotonin, leading to increased anxiety and insomnia—both symptoms of a Busy Brain.

Sugar impacts serotonin production in your gut—the small intestine. In fact, 90% of your serotonin is produced in the gut. If the function of your gut is compromised from overloading it with too much sugar, you'll have trouble with important gut functions like digestion, immune cell formation, and serotonin production.

A high amount of sugar can also impact your brain's ability to produce and utilize serotonin over time. The entire series of B vitamins—especially folic acid—is essential for the production of serotonin. A high-sugar diet forces your body to use up its B vitamins to metabolize sugar, leaving low levels of the various forms of vitamin B for the production of serotonin or other important functions in the brain.

The impact sugar has on anxiety has a lot to do with how it affects your blood glucose levels. Consuming sugar initiates a blood sugar roller coaster that can feel like an anxiety attack. When blood sugar levels crash, the brain becomes desperate for energy, and your body can become shaky, weak, confused, and anxious in your hypoglycemic state (another name for "low blood sugar"). As blood sugar levels plummet, the brain reacts by sending out a panicked adrenaline alarm, leading to anxiety.

In addition, when you eat foods that raise your blood sugar level, the amount of a protein called brain-derived neurotrophic factor (BDNF) decreases. BDNF plays a vital role in reducing anxiety, panic, and stress reactions, so a deficiency can exacerbate Busy Brain symptoms.

So, bottom line, consuming high glycemic foods will spike

your blood sugar and cause multiple issues to occur in the brain and the gut with an elevated blood sugar level. These patterns of inflammation in the body and neuroinflammation in the brain fuel many symptoms, including anxiety, difficulty focusing, and insomnia, seen in a Busy Brain.

Aunties are doing a facepalm here. "Hai hai, what am I going to serve when company comes over for chai in the afternoon? I just ordered the fancy tea biscuits from Harrods. What about after serving spicy haleem and biryani for dinner? No good hostess would refuse. Dessert after a heavy, spicy meal is a basic hosting duty."

Let me be clear, this is going to be controversial: I am not against sugar/high glycemic index foods/caffeine, and I will not put you on a low-carb diet. In section three, I will give you the brainSHIFTs to help curb the cravings and introduce you to slow-carb foods. Slow-carb foods are low glycemic index foods; this means foods that contain carbohydrates but do not spike your blood sugar. Examples of slow carbs are brown rice and sweet potatoes. We will break down the entire eating system in weeks 5 and 6 of the brainSHIFT Protocol, and believe it or not, comfort foods are still allowed. (I'll continue to make that promise throughout the book.)

How? Well, we find that once neuroinflammation is calmed down by restoring balance in your circadian rhythm in weeks 1 through 4, people are sleeping better and have less anxiety. Thus, stress eating minimizes, and we stop bingeing foods like cookies, potato chips, and pizza. You will learn that once we have restored balance and stress eating has ceased, we have a system inside the brainSHIFT Protocol that allows you to eat comfort foods.

Sugar in Your Coffee and Cola Is Toxic for Your Brain Cells

Whether it's cookies with afternoon tea, bagels with morning iced coffee, or a croissant with an espresso, so many of us have a habit of quickly grabbing what feels like a one-two punch of energy for our brain. We intensify our sugar cravings when we consume caffeine. Another food group (for so many consider this a food group, though it's not) that can spike insulin levels, causing you to crave high glycemic foods, is caffeine.

As we discussed above, elevated sugar levels in your brain promote inflammation that will depress serotonin levels, which are key to modulating sleep and calming anxiety. When we combine both caffeine and white sugar, we overload the Busy Brain circuits, leading to worsening anxiety and attention deficit. The result? You'll feel more anxious and self-critical over the to-do list that has not been tackled.

But wait, don't panic, I am not taking away caffeine either. In the brainSHIFT Protocol, we create a system for when to have high glycemic carbohydrates, and when to consume caffeine.

Caffeine Focuses a Busy Brain

Now remember, both Aunties and readers, I'm not anti-caffeine as a brain doctor. Caffeine is a stimulant and the most commonly used drug in the world (not only by those of us who love our chai). Every day, millions consume it to increase wakefulness, alleviate fatigue, and improve concentration and focus.

Caffeine has a double-ringed molecular structure similar to that of adenosine, making it a competitive antagonist to adenosine. Adenosine is an inhibitory neurotransmitter in the brain, and acts as a central nervous system depressant to help us feel calm and regulate sleep. As the day progresses, adenosine binds to its receptors in the brain, causing drowsiness. However, when caffeine binds to these adenosine receptors, it blocks the binding of adenosine. Therefore, instead of feeling drowsy, with caffeine your brain can now maintain a state of vigilance, focus, and energy.

In prescription and over-the-counter (OTC) medicines, caffeine is used to treat tiredness and drowsiness and improve some pain relievers' effects. It belongs to a group of drugs called central nervous system (CNS) stimulants. Foods containing caffeine can help restore mental alertness. Caffeine's use as an alertness aid should only be occasional, and it is not intended to replace sleep and should not regularly be used for this purpose. We must be mindful of how much caffeine we consume, and when.

In the United States, more than 90% of adults use caffeine regularly, with an average consumption of more than 400 mg of caffeine per day. This is more caffeine than in two 6-ounce cups of coffee or five 12-ounce cans of soft drinks. The recommended dose of caffeine is typically less than 200 mg daily.

How do you know if you have too much caffeine? You may want to cut back if you're drinking more than four cups of caffeinated coffee a day (or the equivalent) and you have side effects such as headache, insomnia, increased anxiety, nervousness, irritability, frequent urination, inability to control urination, fast heartbeat, or muscle tremors.

When is the right time to drink caffeine? Do you make a cup the first thing when you wake up? If your Busy Brain score was higher than 30, you might need that energy boost. However, when we are healthy without neuroinflammation, our cortisol levels are naturally highest in the morning, so know that drinking coffee immediately after waking up may decrease its energizing effects, as your stress hormone cortisol is at its peak level at this time.

It is normal for cortisol to be elevated in the morning, and in normal circumstances, it is a hormone that can enhance alertness and focus. It also regulates your metabolism, immune system response, and blood pressure.

The hormone cortisol follows a rhythm specific to your sleep-wake cycle, that is, your circadian rhythm. In the absence of neuroinflammation, cortisol levels peak 30 to 45 minutes after you rise and slowly decline throughout the rest of the day. That said, it has been suggested that the best time to drink coffee is mid- to late morning, when your cortisol level is lower.

For most people who get up around 6:30 a.m., this time is between 9:30 and 11:30 a.m.

If you drink coffee later in the day, it can impair your circadian rhythm and disturb sleep. Remember that even if the energizing effects of caffeine have worn off, the stimulating effects of caffeine from coffee last 3 to 5 hours, and depending on individual differences, about half of the total caffeine you consume remains in your body after 5 hours. You will see in the brainSHIFT Protocol we try to cut caffeine out after 1:00 p.m. to restore harmony with sleep and circadian rhythm. So essentially, your caffeine time if you wake at 6:30 a.m. would be between 9:30 a.m. and 1:00 p.m.

Before you set your clocks, know that there is evidence that caffeine may impair insulin action, leading to a small but detectable rise in blood sugar levels, particularly after meals. If your meal contains high glycemic index foods (sugar), you are now increasing the risk of spiking blood sugar levels, requiring more insulin.

When we think of the hormone insulin, we think of regulating blood sugar—but it's also an essential part of brain function. Insulin helps maintain the health and growth of brain cells. As more dietary sugar is consumed, the hormone insulin becomes less effective. As your blood sugar becomes more and more elevated, the brain becomes even more resistant to the essential actions of insulin. And as the brain becomes numb to the actions of insulin, your ability to focus and other cognitive functions decline. In a study that followed over 5,000 participants over the course of a decade, researchers found that people with high blood sugar had significantly faster rates of cognitive decline—and the higher the sugar, the swifter the decline.

Clinical studies on people with type 2 diabetes report that blood glucose levels rise after consuming caffeine. Additional studies show that with excessive caffeine intake, even individuals without a diagnosis of diabetes can see a spike in insulin levels—creating a drop in blood sugar, causing you to crave sugar.

In summary, I began this conversation with a story of comfort food and how we embrace that in the brainSHIFT Protocol. However, we do need to control stress eating. As you've seen, I am not against high glycemic foods. I am not against caffeine either, but it has to be consumed in the right amount and in the right time for your peak performance. In section three, you will see how we help you to manage the timing of consuming carbohydrates—preferably slow carbs (low glycemic carbohydrates). And you will find out how we manage to schedule your caffeine intake separately from sugar (high glycemic foods). These are the brainSHIFTs that allow you the liberty to eat the foods you desire but in a certain order.

Let me clarify. I am not asking you to detox or cleanse. In fact, I promised at the beginning of this book that comfort foods like angel food cake are celebrated, while brainSHIFT will curb your stress eating.

When I look back now, I appreciate how even with a very full schedule, Dr. Pritchard took the time to teach all of us resident physicians, including those of us like me who needed additional mentoring in the "angel food cake factor." I met him at a time when having a female physician in neurology was rarer than finding a chicken tikka masala recipe in Charleston. Dr. Pritchard was a true model of a STEMinist, mentoring and sponsoring female leaders like myself in a traditional medical system and specialty that did not have many women physicians or leaders. From Dr. Pritchard, I not only started my passion for treating epilepsy patients but also learned some basic tenets of writing a research paper.

At the end of every monthly rotation, Dr. Pritchard and his gracious wife, Becky, would invite the team to dinner in their home. I knew from my traditional South Asian upbringing that this was a big honor—and to replace my smelly hospital scrubs with silk and pearls. But none of that mattered around their dinner table as we savored his famous homemade Pritchard Pesto on seared scallops—and got to share our "angel food cake factor" moments with his family.

Most importantly, from Dr. Pritchard, I officially learned the Southern tradition of comfort food and came to understand that all cultures have their own version. It is with a sense of grief I share that while I was in the process of editing this book, Dr. Pritchard lost his battle to pancreatic cancer in May 2023 on his 80th birthday. I use many of his leadership lessons in my role as a female founder and Chief Wellness Officer. Being able to pause and talk about comfort food has been a bonding experience for me as a Chief Wellness Officer at Evolution Hospitality. With hotels in the United States and Canada, we have a global and diverse workforce. My property tours remind me of attending rounds with Dr. Pritchard; I know that my colleagues at Evo are nervous that a brain doctor and leader from corporate has arrived on the hotel property. Little do they know how nervous I am too, but put a meal in front of us—or get us talking about favorite comfort foods—and we are all relieved. They are relieved that the company physician is not putting them on a diet, and I'm relieved that I can be their Dr. Auntie Romie, making them feel cared for in an organization that puts the well-being of their employees as a top priority.

brainDUMP Chapter 7 Summary

- You do not have to give up comfort foods to cure your Busy Brain.

- There is a difference between comfort foods and stress eating.

- Comfort foods are tied to culture, memories, ancestors, and holidays—and bring joy.

- Stress eating is fueled by a Busy Brain to bring calm to a frazzled nervous system by craving sugars, salts, and carbohydrates.

- High glycemic foods spike your blood sugar, which not only is bad for daytime energy but also fuels neuroinflammation, making a Busy Brain worse.

- Your stress eating is not your fault. Disruption of your circadian rhythm fuels inflammation in the body, which creates your cravings.

- Be a STEMinist—support the young girls and women in your life in an education and career in science, technology, engineering, math, and medicine.

quickSHIFT: Take Fast Action Now

We love to learn about the favorite comfort foods of our global #brainSHIFT community. You can log on to *www.*

BusyBrainCure.com or the brainSHIFT app and share your comfort food.

You can also find Dr. Pritchard's famous homemade pesto sauce recipe and the comfort recipes of many of my loved ones in appendix C.

8

Food and Fat as brainFUEL for a Busy Brain

Sitting down to Pritchard Pesto over seared scallops, angel food cake, and sweet tea at their gracious home, I felt as if I was with my Auntie and Uncle, being offered comfort for working 4 weeks straight without a peaceful night of sleep. At that time in my life, the sweet tea and my ambition for my career kept me moving forward, and I didn't give much thought to the sleep deprivation that was a regular part of residency training in medicine.

We were brainwashed in medical school and during our training to believe that sleep was for the weak. And if I was going to hang with the boys in neurology, I could not let a single bead of sweat or weakness show—including how tired I was. My ego and fragility weren't allowed in medical training, but deep down I feared failure every single day. Even larger was the burden of knowing that failure was not an option. If I were to fail, I was not only letting down my Nanni, mother, Aunties, and our ancestors. I was also letting down my whole gender, for I was acutely aware that at that time, less than 5% of brain doctors in the country were women. I felt that any failure on my part would affect women in medicine for generations to come. Thankfully, Dr. Pritchard and his colleagues in my residency training understood, as fathers of daughters, that diversity was needed in medicine, and they were doing something about it.

At that dinner, Dr. Pritchard put down his fork and turned to me. "I know you just came off the in-patient rotation, but you should switch assignments to be the resident physician on the wards again starting tomorrow. Dr. Braxton B. Wannamaker III will be the attending physician this month."

I stopped stuffing my face with the delectable Southern comfort food and immediately understood the assignment. Dr. Wannamaker needed no introduction in the medical world. He was a legend who walked the halls of the Medical University of South Carolina (MUSC). (Sorry, not sorry, Dr. Wannamaker. I know with your humility you'll be mortified to read this.) He was not only a full professor of neurology and the past president of the American Epilepsy Society, but he had also dedicated his career to cutting-edge research in antiepileptic medications and sudden unexpected death in epilepsy. I wanted to learn from not only his experience with epilepsy patients, but the wisdom of his impact-driven clinical research.

As I took a bite of the soft, pillowy angel food cake, I had a talk with myself at the table. *Girl, raise your hand and say yes, sleep can wait another month. It's another professor with Roman nu-*

merals preceding the MD. You are getting the chance of a lifetime for your career. Do. NOT. Blow. It.

Sleep and sanity be damned, I was back in the neurology wards by 4:00 a.m. the next morning to beat everyone there and make sure I knew the details of every single patient, "angel food cake factors" included. I skipped sensible hospital scrubs for Sunday silk, skirt, and shiny shoes. *Be poised, polished, and professional even if you are frazzled, girl.* I ensured every intern and medical student on the team was also prepped and polished. This was game day. Dr. Wannamaker would arrive at 9:00 a.m., and as the senior resident neurologist on the ward, I wanted to show him that everything was under control. Even the nurses who were cheering on "ThatGirl-Doctor" were polishing up their nurses' stations and giving me a thumbs-up.

Just then, my pager shrilled, and I saw the same words that were on the beeper were simultaneously on the overhead intercom with a booming voice: "Code blue room 717 neurology ward, repeat, code blue room 717 neurology ward…"

Oh, help me, God. That is my floor. One of my patients is either in cardiac or respiratory arrest.

I tried to calm my nervous brain as I ran through the hospital ward by reminding myself that I'd done this before. One of the nurses yelled, "Where is ThatGirlDoctor?" A trail of interns and medical students ran behind me.

I arrived short of breath at the bedside of an elderly woman who was admitted the night prior with stroke-like symptoms. I looked at the heart monitor. She was in atrial fibrillation with rapid ventricular response. She had a dangerous heart rhythm that was unable to pump enough oxygenated blood to organs like her brain and lungs. She was now unable to breathe and was in a coma.

I got through the first steps with a team of our brilliant nurses at my side, secured her airway and breathing, and checked that we still had access to her veins with an intravenous needle to give medication.

And then I froze.

Or choked. Take your pick.

I had memorized those ACLS guidelines for emergencies just like this. Backwards and forwards. ACLS stands for advanced cardiac life support, and these are guidelines designed to simplify quick and efficient treatment for a patient that is having an emergency affecting their heart. This was not my first code blue when I'd needed to use the ACLS guidelines. But they were locked away in my brain, and it was not allowing my memory to access the next steps.

With firm encouragement, one of the nurses yelled, "Come on, Dr. M. You got this. What do we do next?"

But despite the encouragement and cries for help from the nurses, I was still frozen when one of my physician colleagues from the critical care team arrived with his team to help take over. I stepped outside the room to catch my breath and saw Dr. Wannamaker III with his signature bow tie rapidly coming around the corner toward me.

If you are not in medicine, let me spell out this scenario. An attending physician, meaning Dr. Wannamaker III, does not want to walk into work first thing in the morning to a patient he hasn't ever met coding, and to top off that nightmare, to see a petrified senior resident standing outside the door, sweating through her silk.

In traditional Southern gentleman style, he extended his hand and calmly rolled out in a drawl, "Good mornin'. I'm Dr. Wannamaker, the neurology attendin' physician…"

I kept shaking his hand and started to blurt out, "Sir, we have a 72-year-old female admitted overnight with stroke-like symptoms who now is in…"

Cutting me off, he took a breath and said, "My name is Dr. Wannamaker. Hello. May I ask your name?"

I was confused. "Um, Dr. Mushtaq. I mean, my first name is Romila. But no one other than my Aunties can pronounce that, so the whole world knows me as Romie."

He nodded his head. "Oh, Rohmillah like vanilla…"

"Sir, I think I am more caramel than vanilla," I blurted out while inspecting my skin.

Shit! Insubordination along with failing to do my job correctly in a life-threatening situation. I am definitely going to get fired now, and I haven't even finished my residency training. I have no other life or job skills other than medicine. No one will employ me, not even the Chick-fil-A downstairs. I am going to starve and most of all bring shame to my Aunties… Oh good God, what would I even say to my father, Dr. Mushtaq Sr., the cardiologist?

My brain was no longer frozen. Instead, it was spiraling out of control.

Dr. Wannamaker chuckled, and in a matter of seconds, with his calm and gentle reserve, he guided me back into the room. We rejoined the medical team in helping to stabilize our patient and transferred her to the critical care unit.

Typically, in a moment like this in our current toxic medical system, an attending physician like Dr. Wannamaker would not only have the right but would be expected to dress down, threaten, and humiliate me for failing to know a basic life-saving protocol. In front of everyone. Even the nurses who were always cheering on "ThatGirlDoctor" were bracing for his wrath.

Instead, he looked at the rest of our team and told them to go take a break and check on the other patients. Then he peered at me. I was ready to break down into sobs.

"Why don't we go downstairs to the physician's lounge and get a cup of coffee? Paul told me that you are passionate about epilepsy." Dr. Wannamaker shifted the entire scene not only in that moment, but for the rest of my career.

And for you who are not fashion queens who missed one of the key moments in this story, silk and sweat are a funky combination. When the moment counts in your life, leave the stuffy silk fabrics behind. Sorry, Aunties, but you know that is the truth.

brainSCIENCE Break

As I became immersed in learning more about epilepsy and brain health as a resident neurology doctor, I was introduced to the ketogenic diet for children with severe epilepsy. Children with refractory epilepsy have seizures that continue despite multiple medications. The ketogenic diet for epilepsy patients is very different from the trendy ketogenic diet fad of today. For epilepsy syndromes such as infantile spasms, Rett syndrome, tuberous sclerosis complex, and Dravet syndrome, to name a few, a ketogenic diet is prescribed by a physician and closely monitored by a trained nutritionist. My point is that it was during this time of being introduced to the ketogenic diet that I first became curious about the role of nutrition to keep a brain healthy, and more answers about the benefits of nutrition came when I added my integrative medicine training to my knowledge base.

I made a promise at the outset of this book that I would not put you on a diet or cleanse. As a Chief Wellness Officer for a large company, I want vegans, ketogenic diet followers, paleo, the anti-diet crowd, and everyone else to sit at one table and feel like they belong.

However, I will not dispute the mounting medical evidence that the Mediterranean diet is superior in protecting brain health against aging, stroke, and cognitive decline.

But I also live in the real world, working with professionals who travel, eat out, and have full lives. Meal prep is not possible for everyone, nor is sticking to a strict regimen when dining at restaurants for business client dinners.

So in section three, you will see the biohacks for nutrition that are easy to follow whether you eat in your kitchen, grab a quick bite on the way to the subway, or are connecting through the ATL B concourse and enter the Delta Sky Club. (Say hi to Rondah if you see her.)

Fats Are Not the Enemy for Your Brain

Nutrition advice about what to eat is absolutely confusing, is chaotic, and creates further anxiety around eating. I want to start with one key statement, regardless of what type of nutrition plan you follow (or don't follow). Fats are NOT the enemy. Period.

Not all fats are created equal. Believe it or not, your functioning brain is primarily made up of fat molecules called phospholipids. And in addition, to keep functioning, your brain needs fat to feel fueled. Now, this is not a hall pass to bust out the cast-iron skillet and toss in a pound of butter to fry up some bacon. I'm going to ask you to hit the pause button because there is a difference between healthy and not-so-healthy fats.

The root cause of Busy Brain symptoms is a specific pattern of inflammation that disrupts your brain cell functions of how cells communicate and how effectively molecules can attach to receptors. To calm neuroinflammation that causes a Busy Brain, your brain needs key nutrients such as healthy fats. Here is a challenge I face when teaching the cure to the Busy Brain. It can be confusing what type of fats are "good" for the brain, and what type of fats are not so healthy for the brain and body. The difference in clinical nutrition terms is what we call unsaturated fats (good fats) and saturated fats (not-so-healthy fats).

Omega-6 vs. Omega-3 Fatty Acids

Several sources of information suggest that human beings evolved on a diet with a 1:1 ratio of omega-6 to omega-3 essential fatty acids (EFAs), whereas in Western diets, the ratio is 15:1 to 16.7:1. Western diets are deficient in healthy omega-3 fatty acids and have excessive amounts of the unhealthy omega-6 fatty acids.

Excessive amounts of omega-6 polyunsaturated fatty acids (PUFAs) and a very high omega-6:omega-3 ratio, as is found in today's Western diets, promote the pathogenesis of many diseases, including cardiovascular disease, cancer, and inflammatory and autoimmune diseases.

Increased levels of omega-3 PUFAs (a low omega-6:omega-3 ratio) exert anti-inflammatory effects in the brain and in the heart. When we review the medical data and try to find the right ratio to prevent disease, it is found that:

- A ratio of 4:1 was associated with a lower risk and prevention of cardiovascular disease.

- A ratio of 4:1 was also associated with a 70% decrease in total mortality (risk of death from heart disease).

- A ratio of 2.5:1 reduced the growth of cancer cells in patients with colorectal cancer.

- The lower omega-6:omega-3 ratio in women with breast cancer was associated with decreased risk.

- A ratio of 2:1 to 3:1 suppressed inflammation in patients with rheumatoid arthritis, and a ratio of 5:1 had a beneficial effect on patients with asthma, whereas a ratio of 10:1 had adverse consequences.

These studies indicate that the optimal ratio may vary with the disease under consideration. Therefore, it is quite possible that the therapeutic dose of omega-3 fatty acids will depend on the degree of severity of the disease resulting from the genetic predisposition. A lower ratio of omega-6:omega-3 fatty acids is more desirable in reducing the risk of many of the chronic diseases of high prevalence in Western societies, as well as in developing countries, that are being exported to the rest of the world.

According to *The Blue Zones Solution* by Dan Buettner, food quality was one consistent factor in the five places in the world—dubbed blue zones—where people live the longest and are healthiest. These blue zones are Okinawa, Japan; Sardinia, Italy; Nicoya, Costa Rica; Ikaria, Greece; and Loma Linda, California. While there are many factors involved in these regions' longevity, one consistent theme was a healthier ratio of saturated to polyunsaturated fats, near 1:1. A similar ratio of fats is seen in the Mediterranean diet.

Omega-3 Fatty Acids Fight Neuroinflammation

Among the fatty acids, it is the omega-3 polyunsaturated fatty acids (PUFAs) that possess the most potent anti-inflammatory and immune-boosting activities in the brain. There are three types of omega-3 PUFAs: eicosapentaenoic acid (EPA) and docosahexaenoic acid (DHA), and alpha-linolenic acid (ALA). Both EPA and DHA types of omega-3 fatty acids are more potent than ALA.

The functions of omega-3 fatty acids include regulation of the amount and types of eicosanoids made. In addition, other effects are elicited by eicosanoid-independent mechanisms, including actions upon intracellular signaling pathways, transcription factor activity, and gene expression.

The eicosanoids formed play important roles in brain function including:

1. Sleep induction (PGD2)

2. Cognitive and executive function, specifically long-term potentiation, spatial learning, and synaptic plasticity (PGE2)

3. Healing and resolving neuroinflammation (lipoxins)

4. Anti-inflammatory and neuroprotective bioactivity (dihydroxy-docosatriene, neuroprotectin D1, formed from DHA)

So, in summary, healthy polyunsaturated fats play a crucial role in aspects of daytime cognition, including learning and attention span. They also help to regulate sleep. And lastly, they battle neuroinflammation.

Dr. Claudia Satizabal and her research team published a 2022 study of 2,183 healthy volunteers who did not have any signs, symptoms, or history of dementia or stroke. The average age of the study participants was 46 years old. The study showed:

1. Higher omega-3 index was associated with larger hippocampal volumes. The hippocampus, a structure in the brain, plays a major role in learning and memory.

2. Consuming more omega-3s was associated with better abstract reasoning, or the ability to understand complex concepts using logical thinking.

3. APOE4 carriers with a higher omega-3 index had less small-vessel disease. The APOE4 gene is associated with cardiovascular disease and vascular dementia.

Coronary heart disease, major depression, aging, and cancer are characterized by an increased level of interleukin-1 (IL-1), a pro-inflammatory cytokine. Similarly, arthritis, Crohn's disease, ulcerative colitis, and lupus erythematosus are autoimmune diseases characterized by a high level of IL-1 and the pro-inflammatory leukotriene LTB4 produced by omega-6 fatty acids.

There have been a number of clinical trials assessing the benefits of dietary supplementation with fish oils in several inflammatory and autoimmune diseases in humans, including rheumatoid arthritis, Crohn's disease, ulcerative colitis, psoriasis, lupus erythematosus, multiple sclerosis, and migraine headaches. Many of the placebo-controlled trials of fish oil in chronic inflammatory diseases reveal significant benefits, including decreased disease activity. All of these diseases have an increased level of IL-1 in common. An elevation of pro-inflammatory cytokines, including IL-1, is also seen in symptoms of a Busy Brain (as we discussed in chapter 6).

In a standard diet promoting low-fat consumption, fat intake is unbalanced. Low omega-3 polyunsaturated fatty acids (n-3 PUFAs) have been associated with neuropsychiatric and neurological disorders with inflammation, including ruminating anxiety, ADHD, and insomnia. Yes, one of the unwanted side effects of decades of a low-fat diet is creating symptoms of a Busy Brain. In addition to fueling your brainPOWER, consuming healthy fats will also reduce your harmful belly fat.

Leptin signals your brain that you are full and should stop eating. Leptin also supports efficient metabolism. If too much leptin builds up in your blood, you may develop leptin resistance. When this occurs, the leptin in your body may not do its job effectively, resulting in weight gain. The mechanisms that can cause leptin to build up in your bloodstream? You guessed it—sleep deprivation, stress, and a Busy Brain. Cortisol, one of the hormones that is elevated when you have a Busy Brain, may make your brain less receptive to leptin and cause you to overeat.

The conclusion, if you have a Busy Brain, is that your elevated stress hormones may be blunting your ability to lose weight. Eating healthy fats is one of the key nutrition recommendations for restoring your leptin levels (in addition to sleep). By the end of weeks 5 and 6, 60% of our participants reported reduced belly bloating, a drop in pants/dress size, and losing weight. Most importantly, they report feeling fueled without energy highs and lows throughout the day.

Methylation Disorders

While we are on the topic of getting fueled and energized throughout the day, it would be unwise to ignore a group of genetic disorders. In both my previous clinical practice and taking clients through the 8-week brainSHIFT Protocol, I have consistently diagnosed methylation disorders during our routine laboratory evaluations.

Now, you don't need to run and grab a 23andMe kit or start hunting down your ancestry to see if any of your Aunties are responsible for your Busy Brain. While many genetic diseases can affect the brain and mental health, the one key issue I screen for is methylation disorders. Under this category, the most common is the methylenetetrahydrofolate reductase (MTHFR) mutation.

MTHFR produces an essential enzyme that converts folate

into a form that plays a role in mood-regulating neurotransmitter production. If you find out that you have the MTHFR mutation, do not let your Busy Brain create panic. This diagnosis is an opportunity to change your diet and lifestyle to maximize your methylation, manage symptoms, and optimize your overall health.

When an MTHFR mutation occurs, there is a risk of elevated markers of neuroinflammation and inflammation in the body. MTHFR deficiency is the most common genetic cause of elevated levels of homocysteine in the plasma (hyperhomocysteinemia) and reduced levels of folic acid in the blood. While there are many risks associated with the MTHFR mutation, from cardiovascular disease to increased risk of miscarriages, two important medical problems linked to this deficiency are anxiety and attention deficit disorder.

The MTHFR enzyme plays an essential role in processing amino acids, specifically converting homocysteine to methionine. Methionine is an essential amino acid that is required to build proteins in the body.

We routinely screened for these disorders when I was in neurology practice assessing risks of heart disease, stroke, and abnormal clotting. However, as I deepened my knowledge in integrative medicine, I learned the clinical research also showed that methylation disorders are a root cause of brain and mental health disorders such as depression, attention deficit disorder, and anxiety.

The treatment is simple. We check homocysteine levels, and if they are high, we treat them with folic acid. There is solid clinical evidence that methylfolate (also known as L-methylfolate,

5-MTHF, or 5-methyltetrahydrofolate) is a biologically active form of folate, so it is easier for your body to absorb.

As I look back at my first meeting with Dr. Wannamaker, it's easy to see that I had a Busy Brain, and even his invite for a coffee in the physician's lounge still had me assuming the worst. I worried that I had failed, and as you know, for me, failure was not an option. But ultimately, I didn't fail. I went on to have a successful career guided by my mentors.

When I decided to leave traditional neurology and pursue a career in integrative medicine, initially it was difficult for me to face Drs. Wannamaker and Pritchard. I felt like I was disappointing them as they had trained me to grow up and be a full professor in neurology who created an impact for epilepsy patients—just like they had. In 2018, I saw both of them together at Dr. Wannamaker's home in South Carolina. By this time, I was well into my role as Chief Wellness Officer at Evolution Hospitality and was busy scaling my business. As we sat over a traditional Southern Christmas dinner on his family's fine china, I realized that I was already honoring them as my career mentors and sponsors—by taking their lessons of compassion, connection, and now comfort food forward in my role as a leader. I also know that I couldn't have written this book or completed the research around Busy Brain without every skill they had taught me over 20 years ago. When we have a teacher of compassion, we not only find healing but also a path forward on our own unique terms.

It's also funny that when we are sleep-deprived and have a Busy Brain, we remember the worst of ourselves. Dr. Wannamaker didn't remember that we met over a patient nearly dying. He simply remembered taking me under his wing because I was a daughter of a doctor, and he too had a daughter that he hoped would enter medicine one day. He was acutely aware that the current system needed to improve to welcome women in medicine and that by guiding me, someone would one day be there to guide his daughter.

And you better believe, until this day, I have never forgotten the ACLS guidelines to treat atrial fibrillation with a rapid ventricular rate. When I wake up in the middle of the night spiraling, to make sure I am okay, I recite the protocol to make sure I am still in control. It not only helps guide me back to sleep, but it soothes my heart.

brainDUMP Chapter 8 Summary

1. Healthy fats are fuel for your brain, weight management, and performance.

2. A ratio of unhealthy fats (omega-6) to healthy fats (omega-3) is ideal at 1:1, but even reducing it to 4:1 has clinical benefits for the brain and physical health. Current standard Western diets average a ratio of 16:1.

3. Healthy fats are called healthy fats because they are essential to your brain structure and function. In addition, none of our body's fifty hormones can be created or work without healthy fats.

9

Technology and a
Busy Brain

Beats of hip-hop music pulsated on the other side of the door as I paused, trying to summon the courage to enter the corporate headquarters of Evolution Hospitality. My chest spasmed almost as quickly as the rhythm of the music, and I struggled to swallow the saliva pooling at the back of my throat—a telltale sign that my stress levels were high enough to trigger my achalasia symptoms.

Here I was, a geek girl with frizzy hair, about to make a ridiculous ask of the president of a company whose operations run 24 hours a day, 7 days a week, 365 days a year. I took a deep breath and practiced my ask one last time: "I'd like for all of your employees to stop working and shut down emails, phones, and all digital devices 1 hour before bedtime. And then I want to collect data about their brains."

Practicing wasn't helping my nerves, and my Busy Brain immediately clicked to "hyperdrive mode." I spiraled down a rabbit hole of self-doubt and judgment. Whenever I got lost this deep into hyperdrive Busy Brain mode, my mother's and Aunties' judgmental voices were always front and center. *"We were right: even though you are a brain doctor, you have lost your mind. You left your esteemed hospital job as a practicing physician to become a—what is it called again—'an entrepreneur'? Hai hai, I don't even know what that means…"*

As soon as I heard their words in my mind, my natural instincts to run to safety kicked in. I was ready to bolt back to my overpriced rental car and drive to the nearest beach in Southern California to ponder whether I could beg for my hospital job back again. Too late. The doors to Evolution Hospitality slid open, and I was snapped out of my obsessive and ruminating brain battle. The loud music snapped me back to present-centered awareness, and I glanced into the room.

The open-spaced office gave off a mixed vibe of sexy bachelor pad and West Coast tech start-up. As I stepped a few more feet into this Cali-cool office, I spied two marketing team members who were battling each other at the ping-pong table with onlookers cheering them on. On the wall behind the ping-pong table was the company's guiding ethos: "It's not how we work, it's how we live."

So, this is where all the cool kids ended up after high school. It's only 8:45 a.m., and the party has already started; wow, how did I get an invitation here? I pulled down my heavy navy wool blazer and glanced at my Jimmy Choos.

Before my brain could head back down my familiar rabbit hole, I was welcomed by the party folks, and I began to see the reality of this people-driven culture. It was as if a small town of family and friends welcomed me. I felt a surge of warmth in my heart, and my achalasia symptoms subsided.

Bulmaro Farias, a director of corporate talent in Human Resources, was already waiting in the kitchen, smiling and offering me a hug and a much-needed frothy cappuccino. Bulmaro had been the first Evo employee to see my TEDx talk on mindfulness and had introduced my mission to his organization 2 years prior. Shortly after that, they'd hired me as a speaker at their leadership conference. I already knew this was a unique and forward-thinking company, but my Busy Brain was still on alert.

Bulmaro could sense my excited nerves and reminded me why I was there with their leadership team. "Evolution spun off from a family-owned business that also had a long legacy of focus on individual well-being, both of mind and body. We invited you into our space because we were ready to evolve beyond traditional education sessions and standard wellness tips. How do we build a systemic wellness culture that is highly interactive and that supports our people toward a better version of themselves?"

I listened, analyzed, and was ready to rehearse my big ask with him. As I took a sip of the caffeine, I noticed a framed quote on the wall showing Evo's wellness triangle. Their wellness triangle was part of their secret sauces and the foundation of their people-driven culture. In the shape of a pyramid, different words were stacked upon each other. At the base of the pyramid shape was the word *sleep*. (My brain doctor's mind approved.) On top of the word *sleep* was written *your calling*. The words stacked above *your calling* were *move* and *nourish*.

On the outside of the pyramid were the words *in the community with loved ones.*

Wow, how did the founders of a hospitality management company figure all of this out? I had gone back to train in integrative medicine and its principles, and yet here was a brilliantly laid out concept of the future of employee wellness based on those same principles. I was standing in a magical moment—*The Universe conspired to bring us together. Maybe they will say yes to my harebrained idea.*

Even before the president of Evolution Hospitality walked through the doors, a noticeable silence spread throughout the living room. As John Murphy, affectionately known to his inner circle as Murph, strode in, his charisma filled the space.

THE WELLNESS TRIANGLE

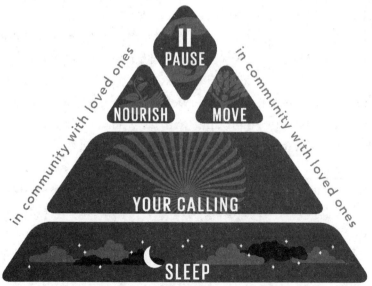

He wore surfer-dude shorts and business shoes but without any socks on. But I knew Murph and not to let his casual appearance and demeanor disarm me. We were in the presence of a visionary leader of a rapidly scaling company with a culture based on the well-being of its employees.

"Rome, hey girl, welcome to San Clemente and Evo's home base," Murph said.

I pulled my gaze away from the wellness triangle to greet him.

Murph then invited me, with my out-of-place stuffy suit, into his office. *Note to self, leave wool and Spanx on the East Coast the next time I visit.* But before I knew it, I'd further outed myself when I took out a binder full of notes I'd overprepared to answer any of the potential legal or HR-related questions of running a clinical study outside of a hospital.

Murph anchored us in his intention for the well-being for Evo's employees. "When we launched the company on 1.1.11 (numbers are important to us) we knew that if we helped our people be the very best version of themselves, they would do exceptional work and our business would grow. And, we believed wholeheartedly in the wellness triangle you were just studying, which we brought with us when leaving Tarsadia Hotels and launching Evolution. We've dabbled with experts in the wellness field. It wasn't until you spoke at our leadership conference last year that we had someone whose credentials and ability to connect with people at a deep level really resonated with a large group of our people."

My Busy Brain shifted into calm consciousness, knowing even more deeply that each one of us in that room had a similar mission to serve our people. Stepping into my authority

THE BUSY BRAIN CURE 173

of medicine, research, and mindful leadership helped me find my voice at that moment.

"The picture of your wellness triangle is a sign from the Universe that I am meant to be here. You all have figured out the path to health that I was not taught as a traditional neurologist. I had to go back for additional training in integrative medicine to learn what you already have in place for your employee wellness. I have ideas on how to use that knowledge to do important research on the Busy Brain while I help you grow your wellness initiatives."

Not exactly the lines I'd practiced, but Murph was in, and I was elated.

We discussed the complex legalities of collecting medical data while making the program a fun wellness challenge for the Evolutionaries, as they're called. A sense of pause came over the three of us in the room. I knew in my mind and, more importantly, in my gut—we were about to plant the seed of something bigger than the three individuals sitting in this room. This moment and idea were bigger than the legacy Murph wanted to leave behind as one of the founders of Evolution Hospitality, and this program would be bigger than my goal of obtaining research data results for this book and future programs.

Little did we know we were about to light the spark—not just for a wellness program but a cultural movement. Thank goodness I didn't drive to the nearest beach and plot to get my old job back. In this moment of flow, both Project Evo and my future role as a Chief Wellness Officer were born.

brainSCIENCE Break

In 2017, as I was starting to unravel the cause of the Busy Brain, I could no longer ignore the role that technology plays in reducing our attention span while simultaneously increasing insomnia. The bottom line is that digital device use at night disrupts our sleep and kills our ability to stay focused and energized during the daytime. I wanted to test how using digital devices and being exposed to blue light at bedtime would impact the daily rhythm of sleep, daytime energy, and attention span. When we stare at the screens of digital devices, including our smart televisions, we are exposed to blue light. This is especially harmful at nighttime. The full light spectrum actually has seven colors, and each of the seven colors in the visible light spectrum has a different wavelength and energy level. Blue light, like that from our digital devices, has a shorter wavelength and higher energy than other colors. Blue light exposure disrupts our circadian rhythm, negatively impacting sleep and attention span.

My theory for the research study was as follows: if we cut out digital device stimulation for 30 to 60 minutes before bedtime, we could quickly reset the employees' circadian rhythms, and we could then measure tangible results to see if digital detox allowed them to sleep peacefully during the night and feel more focused during the daytime. I named the research project and wellness program "Project Evo."

As discussed in chapter 5, circadian rhythms are finely tuned, 24-hour cycles that help our bodies know when to perform essential functions. Light sensed by our eyes is crucial in aligning our circadian rhythms. For most of human history, our circadian rhythms were closely aligned with sunrise and sunset. In today's modern world, we have lost our connection to sunrise and sunset. Instead, the increased use of artificial light and electronics means we are exposed to increasing light when our brains are genetically wired to sense darkness.

While all types of visible light can affect circadian rhythms, blue light has the most significant impact. The blue light signals your brain to wake up when it should be winding down. In one study, as little as 2 hours of exposure to blue light at night slowed or stopped the release of the sleep hormone melatonin. In addition to assessing if sleep could improve with digital detox at night, I also wanted to measure what would happen to their daytime energy and anxiety levels.

The research was now pointing to screen time being associated with not only sleep disturbances but a reduction in attention span and even adult-onset attention deficit disorders (ADHD and ADD). Before our research study at Evolution Hospitality, a study of the impact of digital devices on a Busy Brain had not been done outside the clinical/sleep lab setting.

Your Attention Span Suffers with a Busy Brain

Attention is a topic widely discussed publicly and widely studied scientifically. In its most generic form, attention is merely an overall level of alertness or ability to engage with surroundings. Many people don't know that our attention span is also directly linked to the healthy functioning of our circadian rhythm.

There are three types of attention:

1. Focused attention refers to our ability to focus attention on a stimulus—for example, focusing on an abrupt noise in a quiet room and assessing if you are in danger.

2. Sustained attention is the ability to attend to a stimulus or activity over a long period of time, such as sitting through your fifth team meeting for the day, while avoiding checking for texts or emails on your phone.

3. Selective attention is the ability to attend to a specific stimulus or activity in the presence of other distracting stimuli. For example, this could be maintaining focus on what is happening in that meeting while analyzing the source of that loud noise outside the conference room.

During the course of your day, all three types of attention are needed to conquer your to-do list and optimize performance. When we have a Busy Brain, all three are negatively impacted. Research shows that in today's hyperconnected digital world, your attention span is shorter than that of a goldfish, less than 9 seconds. Does this mean that we are all suffering a societal ADHD?

If you are nodding your head up and down as you read this, you are not alone. According to a research study published by Jessica C. Agnew-Blais, approximately 50% of American adults with ADHD also have an anxiety disorder. Anxiety disorder and attention deficit disorder are intertwined, and it is hard to determine which one came first. Researchers believe there is a brain connection between them. Attention deficit hyperactivity disorder (ADHD) and anxiety disorders frequently occur together. These conditions can exist simultaneously, or ADHD may contribute to the development of anxiety disorder. If you have anxiety, then you're more likely to have attention disorders (hence the term Busy Brain). Note: a trained health professional should complete an evaluation with you before a diagnosis of adult-onset ADHD is assumed.

Technology Induces Adult-Onset Attention Deficit Disorder

Have you already lost your focus in reading this brain-SCIENCE Break? Before you tell yourself that your brain is not wired for medical information, take a look at how many digital devices surround you at work and, more importantly, in the nighttime. For instance, when I am not being mindful, I'm answering emails on my laptop while watching something random on Netflix, and looking at my iPhone to see if that hot guy texted me back (shhh, don't tell my Aunties!).

What does an audit of your digital device use look like, especially 1 hour before you go to bed? Think about your home and the persistent state of being plugged into computers, smartphones, tablets, e-readers, and even smart televisions. Can you pay attention to an entire episode of the latest binge-worthy series without picking up your phone? This is the reality of our modern-day world where constant technology use is mandatory during the day in our jobs or schools, and then in the evening for our social lives and entertainment. On top of that, there is the constant pull to check in on social media platforms and our email inboxes after work.

My Aunties are the only people who still have the luxury of saying no to virtual gatherings. They turn down my offers of virtual chai parties because they still need help figuring out how to use the camera on the smartphone in selfie mode. If I schedule a FaceTime with them, the camera is pointed not to their face but to their lap or unpedicured feet stuffed in crusty house slippers. (In their defense, those house slippers are replaced by formal house slippers that color coordinate with the sofa pillows when you arrive for chai in person.) Aunties aside, the rest of us are required to say yes to answering urgent work emails at night or attending those virtual PTA meetings.

When I started my medical training, I was like my Aunties without a smartphone and still carried around thick medical textbooks. In the late 1990s, I trained under the guidance and leadership of Drs. Pritchard and Wannamaker (whom you met in chapter 8) in a neurology residency. At that time, adult-onset attention deficit disorder (ADD) was not a recognized medical syndrome. If one had attention deficit hyperactivity disorder (ADHD) or ADD as an adult, it was assumed that it had been present in childhood.

Back then, we had paper charts and pagers. Enter any doctor's office or hospital today and multiple digital screens are sitting between you and your provider. Since my smartphone-deprived neurology training days in the late 1990s, there has been increased expansion and use of the internet, video games, smartphones, and screen time in all work and school environments. Now the diagnosis of adult-onset ADD has completely shifted because the research had to advance to take into account the increased use of technology and exposure to screen time.

Researchers from the Institute of Psychiatry, Psychology

THE BUSY BRAIN CURE

and Neuroscience at King's College London found that nearly 70% of young adults with ADHD did not meet the criteria for the disorder at any of the childhood assessments. Adults with this "late-onset" ADHD had high levels of symptoms, impairment, and other mental health disorders. The researchers suggested that "adult ADHD is more complex than a straightforward continuation of the childhood disorder," according to a published study in *JAMA Psychiatry* in 2017.

The predominant features of ADHD in adults differ from typical ADHD features in children. Studies today have found that most adults with ADHD did not have the condition in childhood. Symptoms of hyperactivity or impulsivity are less evident in adults. If adults are impulsive, it is likely more with words and verbalizations than the physical outbursts seen in children. Here is the key, however: symptoms of inattention are more prominent in adults. In addition to difficulty paying attention, mood disruption—specifically anxiety—is a key feature. As you read this, think about the individual on your team constantly interrupting a meeting, often with an inappropriate sidebar or comment that doesn't align with your HR policies. We all know that person, and at times, we can all be that person. Could it be that adult-onset ADHD is a part of a Busy Brain?

Today, as I research and treat teams with Busy Brain, I can no longer ignore the role of technology and our attention span, that is, our ability to focus. ADHD in adults is characterized by symptoms of inattention, impulsivity, and restlessness, resulting in functional impairment. The executive function in your brain, i.e., your ability to analyze and process data, is impaired. Emotional dysregulation—a mood or mental health disorder—is highly likely to coexist with adult-onset ADHD. The two most common mood disorders coexisting with adult-onset ADHD are substance abuse and anxiety. As we look at workplace performance and organizational psychology data, it's no wonder that ADHD in adulthood is associated with significant impairment in studying, work performance, and the ability to socialize.

Project Evo: Digital Detox for an Entire Company

One month after I pitched my research idea to Murph, I returned to Evo's corporate headquarters to officially launch the Project Evo study. Every month, Evo's people come together at their monthly town halls known as "CONNECT meetings." I invited approximately 500 of our leaders in a company of over 5,000 employees to "disconnect to reconnect" and sign up for Project Evo, and 427 raised their hands to join. For this Project Evo wellness and research program, we asked leaders from the corporate office and the hotels they managed to sign up for a 21-day digital detox challenge. By signing up, they committed to turning off their digital devices a minimum of 30 minutes and up to 60 minutes before bedtime. Individuals were given additional options to limit caffeine and alcohol intake but were instructed not to change any dose of medications or supplements they were using.

Before the program started, all 427 participants were asked to take an initial 21-question pretest that measured their stress and energy levels as a baseline assessment. To study if digital detox helps the Busy Brain, it was important for me to understand the baseline sleep issues, anxiety scores, and stress levels in their brains.

The questions for the assessment were derived from validated medical questionnaires: the Pittsburgh Sleep Scale, Workplace Stress Scale, and State-Trait Anxiety Inventory. Of the 427 leaders who signed up for the program, 337 individuals completed the test before starting the Project Evo program. You can read the list of twenty-one questions and the full white paper with the online resources at *www.BusyBrainCure.com.*

The results surprised me and were a wake-up call to Evo's leadership. Despite a people-driven culture and reported happiness at work, the data showed Evolutionaries had low energy getting up in the morning, were stressed at work, and had disturbed sleep. Prior to the start of the 21-day digital detox program, the results of our screening questionnaire revealed the following:

- 48% reported feeling stressed more than half of the workweek.

- 70% reported difficulty falling asleep at night.

- 42% woke up in the middle of the night and could not go back to sleep.

- 75% woke up feeling low on energy and fatigued.

During the program, participants had access to videos on the importance of digital detox, guided meditation, and once-weekly live calls with me discussing self-care while instructing them on how to progress with digital detox each week.

At the end of the 21 days, we asked participants to take the same 21-question assessment. A total of 188 people completed the entire 21-day digital detox. The other individuals who did not complete the program were used as an internal control group known as the Digital Detox (DD) Failed Group. I then used the data on the 188 people who completed the challenge to compare the before and after effects of people who could complete Digital Detox (DD) versus the same parameters in the DD Failed Group.

When you compared the two groups, we had what is known in medical research as statistical significance (p-value < 0.5%) in improvement in the four key areas. In a research study, when you reach statistical significance, it means the results are valid and not by chance alone. The four key areas in which we reached statistical significance are as follows:

Question 1. "I can fall asleep within 30 minutes of going to bed." Of Evolution Hospitality employees, 76% said yes before and 98% answered yes after in the Digital Detox (DD) Group.

Question 2. "I wake up in the middle of the night and have difficulty falling back asleep." Of Evolution Hospitality employees, 92% said yes before digital detox, and 43% after in the DD Group.

Question 3. "I feel nervous or stressed more than 50% of the week." A whopping 96% of people said yes before the program, and that was drastically reduced to 36% in the DD Group.

Question 4. "I wake up with low energy or am tired when I wake up." Of Evolution Hospitality employees, 98% said yes before the digital detox period, and that number was reduced to 44% afterward in the DD Group.

You can see full research results at *www.BusyBrainCure.com*.

The bottom line results: in the employees who completed the 21-day digital detox program, there was a significant improvement in four key symptoms of a Busy Brain.

1. They could fall asleep easily.

2. They would stay asleep and not wake up in the middle of the night.

3. There was improved energy in the morning and the following day.

4. They reported feeling less stressed at work.

With all this data, perhaps you feel like I'm curing your Busy Brain and insomnia and putting you to sleep right here while you read this page. But it was exciting to this Geek Girl. What you can't see in the numbers is the unexpected magic that happened for these participants during that 21-day period. There were a total of four couples who disconnected from their devices and rekindled their romances. More than one couple had reached out to me with that awkward and difficult situation: "What do we do without our iPads/TVs at bedtime?" Those 3 weeks of digital detox had "forced" people to connect with the other humans in their bedrooms.

To this day, the 21-day digital detox is the most talked

about and requested wellness program at Evolution Hospitality. When I share this data in my keynote lectures to other companies, it plants a seed for similar movements to rethink digital device usage, especially before bedtime. In section three, chapter 12, you'll read the transformational story of one of our Evolutionaries, Nancy, and her family. Spoiler alert: to this day, she still practices digital detox and calls her sisters nightly to tell them she loves them.

Why did 3 short weeks of digital detox have such a profound result for individuals as well as the entire team? How is it possible to reset the rhythm of your brain, which no supplement, overpriced mattress, or trendy sleep device can manage?

Let me be like my Aunties, who keep repeating themselves in case I missed the point the first seventeen times. We must address and reassess how technology disrupts our circadian rhythm. In chapter 5, I explained the importance of resetting your circadian rhythm to cure a Busy Brain. I want to expand on how technology influences your 24-hour biological rhythm as it relates to your sleep and daytime ability to focus. Ideally, powering down your digital devices and all of your lights in your home at least 3 hours before bedtime is ideal; however, in the Project Evo study, we found impact occurs as little as 30 minutes before bedtime.

Adults with a Busy Brain not only have sleep disturbances, but also have trouble prioritizing, starting, and finishing tasks. They tend to be disorganized, restless, and easily distracted. Some may even have trouble concentrating while reading. The inability to stay focused and follow through on tasks can derail careers, ambitions, and relationships. Curing a Busy Brain not only restores your well-being but also impacts your personal and professional life.

In chapter 6, we discussed the impact of hormone imbalance in your thyroid gland and a low vitamin D3 level on your Busy Brain, especially adult-onset ADHD. Without addressing our behaviors around technology and screen time, we cannot cure our Busy Brains, even if we balance our hormones.

In 3 weeks of digital detox during Project Evo, we documented marked improvement in restorative sleep, daytime energy, and the ability to stay focused. As a company, Evolution Hospitality learned the importance of taking a pause prior to bedtime by practicing digital detox. In the next section of the book, you'll hear about me becoming their Chief Wellness Officer and the programs we created, including our workplace mindfulness-based wellness program known as the "Power of Pause." Both the "Power of Pause" program and our other wellness programs helped us tame our Busy Brains at work and as a team.

The Project Evo program wrapped up in late 2017, and in early 2018, Murph was deep into succession planning and thinking of his legacy. His vision was that we could walk into corporate headquarters or any Evolution Hospitality–managed hotel and see Evolutionaries prioritizing mindfulness and wellness. As I mentioned in the beginning of this chapter, I had the honor of being given the task and role of Chief Wellness Officer at Evolution Hospitality and carrying this mission forward. I was the first physician put in this type of a role for a corporation in the United States (outside of hospital systems). Murph later explained his visionary idea: "I knew to succeed in this highly competitive industry (third-party hotel management), we would have to hire the best people while keeping their engagement high and our turnover low. You see, our business didn't create anything tangible. We manufactured nothing. We were only as good as our people who help drive the results at our hotels. We needed to be an employer of choice differentiator. We needed something more than a junior human resource leader putting out a clip-art, monthly wellness letter talking about the importance of exercise. I took the bet that if we hired a triple board-certified neurologist as our Chief Wellness Officer and had her connect intimately with our people, we would have something special as an employer, and it would help us to attract, engage, and retain top talent… It worked."

I never could have imagined this moment when I was meditating with my mindfulness teachers in Cambodia or studying for my integrative medicine boards. Who can truly know what the Universe has in store for us when we cure our Busy Brains?

brainDUMP Chapter 9 Summary

- Blue light is emitted from digital devices and LED lights and can disrupt your circadian rhythm.

- A disruption in your circadian rhythm is one of the root causes of a Busy Brain, and that includes the symptoms of adult-onset attention deficit disorder.

- Do at least 30 minutes of digital detox before bedtime, but up to 60 minutes is ideal.

- When you disconnect from digital devices, you are given a chance to reconnect with your loved ones.

- Digital detox before bedtime can improve both your sleep and your daytime attention span.

- The white paper and full research results for Project Evo can be read at *www.BusyBrainCure.com.*

quickSHIFT: Take Fast Action Now

Does your Busy Brain give you 117 rational-sounding reasons to stop an important project before you take the first step? You tried controlled breathing or guided meditation, but you just could not power down your Busy Brain. In section three, chapter 12 of the book, we introduce digital detox as brainSHIFT number 3 inside the brainSHIFT Protocol.

SECTION THREE

The 8-Week brainSHIFT Protocol

10

brainSHIFT Protocol, Week 1
Stating Goals Instead of
Self-Judgments

I pushed myself past my bedtime to share comfort food at a leadership dinner in downtown Dallas—to finally reunite and laugh in person after the COVID-19 lockdown was worth losing 90 minutes of sleep. Just this one time. As we walked back into the hotel from dinner, the minimalist beige lobby had transformed into a vibrant scene full of partying people that overstimulated my senses. I was ready for bed, but the throngs of convention attendees were not.

I attempted to tiptoe in my stilettos to the elevators, only to hear multiple voices yelling across the foyer.

"Dr. Auntie Romie, Dr. Auntie Romie! Come have a drink."

"We want to take a selfie with you, Dr. Romie. Just one."

"Dr. Romie, how are you still walking in those heels?"

Busted. My plan to try to salvage at least some sleep was

thwarted. I turned back toward the lobby as one of the party-goers walked my way to introduce himself and invite me over for a drink.

Wait. Did a grown man really just call me Auntie?

I could hear my Aunties' grating response to this guy as their voices became one with my voice. *"Hooo, haiii. Do not yell at your elders this way, young man. How old do you think I am anyway? I learned from my Aunties to use special expensive face cream their husbands brought them home from France. With the price we pay for those creams, you should be mistaking me for your sister."*

But I simply smiled at him. Being called Auntie was becoming the norm for me. Somewhere between quoting my Aunties and sharing their voices on stages around the country, I had morphed into my elders. These conference attendees weren't the only people who affectionately called me Auntie.

My Busy Brain took a moment to calculate the cost-benefit of losing more sleep and breaking my own rules. Humanity and my heart won. After 2 years of being stuck on Zoom as the only way to interact with the leaders of this company, it was important to me to connect face-to-face in a buzzing room of conference attendees. Plus, I didn't want to go all the way over to my Auntie dark side just yet, as my real Aunties would have just taken an extra banana and mini cheesecake from the buffet, put the snacks in their oversize purses, and gone to bed hours ago.

"Happy to join you, but I'll skip the cocktails. I'm your opening keynote speaker tomorrow morning." I took a seat next to the man from Arkansas (the only way he introduced himself) and looked at their table full of cocktails. "Do you have any sparkling water? I need to skip the cocktails tonight."

They secured and poured the contents of a funky lime-green aluminum can into a highball glass—"Bartlett pear and Asian ginger flavor"—just the holistic and slightly bougie thirst-quencher I needed as I socialized. However, a few moments later, my Busy Brain started to blur, and with the beginnings of double vision, I could see the fine print on the can… "Cheers, betches, 8% alcohol by vol."

Their version of sparkling water included vodka. Ugh. Not only was my sleep plan for that evening hijacked, but now my ability to walk elegantly to the elevator was also in question. The following morning my voice disappeared.

How many times have you mapped out the perfect day to crush your fitness, nutrition, sleep, and mental health goals only to have one of the "betches" derail you? If we assume the best intentions, our Busy Brains are not the enemy. Our Busy Brains really do start each day intending to control the actions that affect the well-being of our brains and bodies.

It's just sometimes betches come along, build acute on chronic stress, lead us to a path of less-than-ideal choices, bring on shame, and then further fuel us down the spiral of a Busy Brain. When my Busy Brain is down that deep rabbit hole, I start hearing the judgmental voices of my Aunties. *"Oof, we raised you to be a lady and not party in a hotel lobby or drink from an aluminum can while wearing your gold jewelry!"*

Do you hear the voice of self-judgment every time you start a wellness program? Whether it is the internalized voices of judgmental Aunties or a jerk that resides in your brain, you are not alone. When we tame our Busy Brains, that voice of judgment, condemnation, and negativity shifts into the voice of wisdom.

Who are these betches I'm referring to? Any person, event, food, beverage, or unprocessed emotion that tempts you away from what you shoulda, coulda, woulda been doing right.

How many times have you labeled yourself a failure because you did not achieve your health goals? We then go back to a replay loop in our minds with the toxic shoulda, coulda, woulda statements.

"What you shoulda done if you had the chance to do it over again..."

"What you coulda done if you had more time, money, fame..."

"What you woulda done if the Universe had aligned..."

In the above story, I shoulda excused myself to go back to the hotel early from dinner. I coulda read the label on the can carefully, said no thank you to anything in a can printed with the word "betches." I woulda been carrying my own water bottle had I planned better.

Welcome to section three of *The Busy Brain Cure*, where you take action using the brainSHIFT Protocol. I know my fellow Busy Brain folks. Perhaps there are some of you who have been reading or listening to (or skimming) the stories, science, and wisdom of my Aunties in the previous two sections of this book, but I'm guessing many of you may have been thinking, Dr. Auntie Romie, get to the point already. I am not judging you if you skipped straight to this section. A Busy Brain creates an anxious urgency to do something immediately so you will feel back in control.

brainSHIFT

When we brainSHIFT, we toss out the shoulda, coulda, and woulda statements and instead focus on one microhabit at a time. When we master one microhabit, we then stack on the next microhabit.

A microhabit feels natural and joyful for you to implement. Habit stacking helps you add one microhabit to the next in an order that naturally builds upon one another.

A brainSHIFT is a particular microhabit that will have the most impact on healing your Busy Brain. I'm often told that my plan skipped discussions of exercise, massage therapy, or any number of other health and healing remedies. Please understand, exercise and self-care rituals are crucial to brain and physical health. My goal with the brainSHIFT Protocol was to give you the steps to take that will cover the most healing ground quickly so that you can get back into your preferred wellness routine. I am also here to tell you that jumping on Amazon to order a supplement or eating avocados for every meal is not creating a lasting cure for your Busy Brain. They become the shoulda, coulda, wouldas in the graveyard of our wellness goals.

I follow the wisdom of my Aunties by sharing stories and their knowledge for a reason—we create a lasting brainSHIFT when we understand how and why we got stuck with a Busy Brain in the first place. The brainSHIFT Protocol is not meant to be another fad diet or wellness app you download in the New Year only to abandon the entire plan once your Busy Brain wins the battle between anxiety versus sleep.

I invite you to take a brainPAUSE to think, feel, and do.

Analyze your data and the scientific facts. Examine your emotions and desires; why do you want to change? Then take action. When we think, feel, and then do, we create a lasting brainSHIFT.

As we go through these next 8 weeks together, I have included stories of individuals who took these actions. I also summarize the scientific background to help you understand why each brainSHIFT is performed in a particular order. I'll also point you back to other chapters in the previous sections so you can read the research and find more details to identify the root cause of your Busy Brain.

These 8 chapters are organized to give you weekly micro-habits, known as brainSHIFTs, to initiate. Yes, you can skim all 8 chapters now, but stop yourself from cherry-picking your favorite brainSHIFT. This program is designed in a specific order that works to cure your Busy Brain. I'll be honest, some days you will feel like you are in a battle with your Busy Brain, and I am here to let you know that my Aunties and I are on your side.

If you're looking for community, we invite you to the brainSHIFT app, where you can join fellow Busy Brains from all over the world who are in the process of brainSHIFT. You can download the app by going to *www.BusyBrainCure.com*.

Do You Have a Busy Brain?

To start, I want to review the symptoms of a Busy Brain that we covered in section one. Has any one of these issues happened to you on a regular basis in the last 2 weeks?

- You need caffeine, an energy drink, or prescription stimulant medication to get you going in the morning?

- Once you get to work, you are still struggling to focus?

- You need another boost of caffeine or something to eat finally to keep going?

- Your to-do list is multiplying faster than you can cross items off?

- You have multiple browser windows open on your multiple screens and have lost focus?

- You manage to get through the day, but you are not quite at the top of your game?

- By the end of the day, your to-do list is longer than when you started?

- You go home (or step away from your home office desk) and need to take the edge off? (Just one glass of wine, a craft beer, or even some overpriced supplement you bought at the request of a social media influencer.)

- You are trying to calm down, but you are wired and tired? All you need is sleep, but when your head hits your pillow, you can't shut off your racing thoughts. Random facts are on a spin cycle in your brain.

The lack of energy in the morning and the inability to focus are adult-onset attention deficit disorders. This low-level feeling of anxiousness builds to ruminating anxiety, which compounds the ADD to kill productivity. The symptoms bleed into your evening and lead to patterns of sleep disruption. All of these symptoms are signs of a Busy Brain, but you know that by now since you have your Busy Brain score. Right? (In case you haven't taken the Busy Brain Test yet, you can go to *www.BusyBrainCure.com* and take the test for free and enjoy all of our additional free resources.)

The problem is not our busy schedules but how our brain processes tasks, emotions, memories, and incoming information 24/7. I researched and created the brainSHIFT Protocol to help you jump off the stress-success cycle and cure your Busy Brain.

The brainSHIFT Protocol is designed as an 8-week process to optimize your well-being in three key stages.

Stage 1: Restoration

During weeks 1 through 4, the microhabits stack up on one another in order for you to fall asleep and stay asleep. Once you improve your sleep, you will start to feel a calming down of ruminating anxiety.

Stage 2: Boost of Energy and Focus

During weeks 5 through 8, now that a restorative foundation is laid out, your body and brain are ready to have your energy systems optimized. We'll cover the simple nutrition biohacks that are the energy blueprint for your brain and body. And I repeat, you are not going on a diet or cleanse, comfort food will still be allowed, but by this time stress eating has been minimized.

Stage 3: Belonging and Community

Individuals can easily complete this program on their own, as they did when I was seeing patients in my integrative medicine practice, or my private executive coaching clients. One additional benefit we found was that by doing this program with a group of people you know (friends, family, colleagues at work), it helped to heal loneliness. I know many of us have professions that required us to master the art of self-studying in college and internships. Creating and sustaining wellness and behavior change are more likely to be anchored in when completed in a community while enjoying positive reinforcement from peers. When we feel a sense of belonging and go through an experience together with others, we feel connected to our goals and each other, and boost team morale.

Your Three Enemies: Resistance. Denial. Projection.

The three defense mechanisms dressed up as your Busy Brain's best friends who will prevent you from digging deeper, doing the work, and facing your fears are resistance, denial, and projection.

- Resistance is defined as, generally, any action in opposition to, defying, or withstanding something or someone.

- Denial is a natural coping mechanism and a conscious refusal to perceive that painful facts exist.

- Projection is a defense mechanism in which unpleasant or unacceptable impulses, stressors, ideas, effects, or responsibilities are attributed to others.

Have you ever felt like you were less than others because of your ruminating negative thoughts, anxious feelings, or anxiety? Our three enemies show up in all of our brains when we are faced with a call to change the way we cope, behave, and act in our day-to-day lives.

- Resistance: your Busy Brain not wanting to sign up for brainSHIFT or not wanting to go to your primary care physician.

- Denial: your Busy Brain believes that your anxiety and symptoms are just your shortcomings as a leader.

- Projection: your Busy Brain thinks that your company is out of bounds to invite a wellness speaker in to discuss anxiety and mental health. The algorithms online may have recommended this book title, and you are wondering if the artificial intelligence has issues instead.

Resistance, denial, and projection could be the names of my Aunties—the judgmental voices in my (and our) head when we have a Busy Brain. Through the brainSHIFTs, they magically transform to voices of hope and wisdom when we decide to cure our Busy Brains. Do you have judgmental voices in your Busy Brain as well? You are not alone. In this section of the book, you are going to meet several individuals who had a Busy Brain and said they had tried everything for sleep, anxiety, or stress management prior to trying the brainSHIFT Protocol.

You will be introduced to Melanie, my developmental editor, who graciously shared her medical background of living a life with purpose and joy. Yet anxiety showed up for an unexplained reason. She had "done everything right" and followed every protocol given to her by her traditional, integrative medicine, and functional medicine physicians. And you'll meet Kelly, who joined the program only because her team members at her company were joining, and brainSHIFT week 7 literally saved her life. At the end of each of these chapters, you have the brainSHIFT of the week outlined for you. It's an honor to be your Dr. Auntie guiding the way and celebrating you as you decide to leave behind the shoulda, coulda, wouldas and start to brainSHIFT.

brainWORK

Each week you will have homework called brainWORK. Your Busy Brain may be tempted to skim all 8 chapters and cherry-pick what feels easy. Don't let your Busy Brain lure you into cutting corners. You didn't achieve your level of professional success overnight; there is not a quick fix for your Busy Brain either. With your to-do list multiplying, 8 weeks may feel like a long battle. All I will ask you for is 3 minutes during the day and 30 minutes at night.

brainWORK Week 1

We are going to approach the brainSHIFTs in two steps this first week.

brainSHIFT Step 1: Take the Busy Brain Test

At the beginning of the book, I invited you to score your Busy Brain. You may also have your Busy Brain score from hearing me speak. If you scored above a 30, you have a Busy Brain. How is a Busy Brain affecting your brain function, mental health, and physical well-being? We are all different. You read in the opening chapters how a Busy Brain fueled my illness, leading to surgery. For others in this book, it has led to difficulty losing weight, dependence on alcohol, or crippling anxiety.

In case you need to take the Busy Brain Test again, you can do so for free by going to *www.BusyBrainCure. com*, where you will find not only the test but also free resources for each of the brainSHIFTs we will lay out in the weeks to come.

Also, the Busy Brain Test is hosted on a HIPAA-compliant server, so your health information is protected and secure. You will be emailed your results and see your score right away when you finish the 20 questions. You will be invited to retake the test in 8 weeks to see how you have improved.

brainSHIFT Step 2: What Is Your Intention or Goal?

I invite you to take a brainPAUSE and imagine:

1. What specific health goal or outcome would you like to achieve at the end of the 8 weeks?

   Be concrete, positive, and specific. Such as, I will see a reduction in my belly bloating, digest food easily, and lose 5 pounds.

   Examples of goals other Busy Brain folks have set are in the app, which you can download by going to *drromie.com/app*.

   Join a community of individuals who are starting the brainSHIFT Protocol with you and share your goal. You can also practice sharing this goal with someone close to you and invite them on the brainSHIFT journey with you.

2. Who could you be as a leader when you brainSHIFT?

   Would you stop the revolving door at your company? Would you cultivate a culture of kindness and gratitude? Would your parenting style shift to calm consciousness and playfulness?

11

brainSHIFT Protocol, Week 2
7-Day Sleep Challenge

When I first met 58-year-old Charles, a 750 mL bottle of gin was his only remaining trusted companion. His marriage of 20 years to the love of his life was on the rocks, and to say he was losing sleep was an understatement.

In July 2021, he showed up to a virtual community master class with me and a group of students. Every quarter, I hold free live online classes for members of our global brainSHIFT community to discuss updates on our research and share new discoveries in our protocols. Charles made an introduction that caused the entire Zoom chat to pause. "Doc, I haven't slept a full night in 30 years, and my Busy Brain Test score is a 93. I've been watching your YouTube videos about insomnia in the middle of the night, and I am glad you are online live right now. Can you help me?"

Charles's health goal was related to his emotional well-being and his relationship with his wife. He was ready to pay to join the virtual 8-week brainSHIFT Protocol. He was starting with the goal that he wanted to become the man he was 20 years prior when they got married. Together, he and his wife were innovative and successful business owners and had scaled a laboratory evaluation company. The company had been the source of their passion and purpose in life. He went on to share that in early 2020, their company was so successful that they were able to sell and fund their retirement dreams of global travel and a life of luxury. Simultaneously, in early 2020, the global pandemic derailed their dreams, leaving them with the nightmare of being homebound, bored, and without purpose.

Charles shared through frustration and tears on that Zoom meeting, "I spent the last 50 years of my life living as an overachiever always looking to the finish line that never arrived. If this was now my finish line, I didn't want to stop the race. I didn't know what to do sitting at home."

He now spent 16 hours a day in online doomscrolling, consuming the daily news headlines with an online community of people who shared his political viewpoints. His mood would shift with the hourly change in headlines, political commentary, or the number of people arguing with his latest Facebook post. He found an online community of other people he had never met in real life but bonded by feeding into each other's Busy Brains and arguing over the news cycle of the hour and staying perpetually sleep-deprived. In addition to sitting at his desk looking at his computer for 14 to 16 hours straight, he also had the news going on his television in the background. He would eventually go to sleep, only to wake up in the middle of the night with an urge to check how many more people had commented on his latest Facebook post, arguing about last night's toxic headlines. He would then pass out on the couch and wake up feeling absolutely exhausted due to a combination of being hungover, still slightly drunk, and sleep-deprived.

When Charles reached week 2 of the 8-week challenge, he started with the one basic brainSHIFT: set a time to stop watching, listening, reading, and arguing over the news simultaneously (this week's brainWORK). Bedtime was going to be 10:30 p.m., and he would wake up at 6:00 a.m. When he woke up in the middle of the night, he would either lie in bed or find something else in the house to do other than to turn to the news. I counseled him and added supplements, 5-hydroxytryptophan (5-HTP) and magnesium glycinate, which helped him immediately sleep 3 to 4 hours straight—something he hadn't achieved since he got married. He knew he was onto something.

During week 2, he got honest about the amount of gin he was consuming and abruptly cut it by half. By the end of the 4 weeks, he was down to one to two glasses of gin in the evening and sleeping 6 hours straight every night.

This wasn't the first time in his adult life he had tapered off heavy drinking, but this was the first time he was forced to face his truth. He had 50-plus years of emotions stuffed inside his brain that he had never expressed, and now, without a job or purpose to keep him busy, he had to face every single one of them. After completing the sleep challenge you will start this week, he then added the steps for week 3 to help process his long ignored emotions.

I'll be honest, when Charles first joined, I didn't realize his comfort food was gin, let alone an entire bottle at night. My Busy Brain started to panic and worry. *This is an educational class, not a medical consultation. How can I get him to the help he needs, while focusing on the other 330 people here?* He assured me he had called a therapist, with whom he had an on-and-off relationship.

By week 4, when we all thought of ourselves as a community of his cheerleaders and he was making progress, his wife of 20 years left him. Paralyzed by grief and determined not to medicate with his old friend gin, he continued the 8-week community journey. Each week he would arrive like an excited Boy Scout ready for a new badge for completing each week's brainWORK. The sense of accomplishment each week gave him purpose, and being celebrated in an online community of other Busy Brained individuals gave him support, despite his grief.

When the 8-week brainSHIFT was completed, for the first time in 30 years Charles was sleeping without distractions or libations. When I checked in with Charles a few months later, he shared, "I'm sleeping through the night, and I only have one cocktail at Olive Garden every Friday night. My wife and I managed our separation, and amicably parted ways. I lovingly helped her settle into her own home in Palm Beach. I reconnected with my estranged brother and my niece, and they are moving to Florida to join me. I am down to 195 pounds from 240 pounds and getting 7 to 8 solid hours of sleep a night."

The brainSHIFT Protocol had not only restored Charles's sleep but also his sanity and sense of connection to the family he had longed to reconnect with. He is now working on how he can mentor other start-up entrepreneurs in the medical technology field. He is also talking to his therapist on a regular basis.

In chapter 5 of section two, I discuss the three types of sleep disturbance we see with a Busy Brain, and Charles had all three types:

1. Difficulty falling asleep at night.

2. Waking up in the middle of the night and unable to go back to sleep.

3. Waking up feeling exhausted and fatigued.

He showed up every Wednesday with the promise to try one brainSHIFT (or microhabit) per week, and he followed the steps I am laying out in these 8 chapters in order. It all starts with the restoration of sleep here in week 2 of the brainSHIFT Protocol.

brainSHIFT

In chapter 5, we talked about a key root cause of Busy Brain being a disruption in your circadian rhythm. The circadian rhythm is key in modulating your sleep-wake cycle. In this week's brainSHIFT, we are going to complete a 7-day sleep challenge that is built on principles of sleep hygiene and cognitive behavioral therapy for insomnia.

For certain clients who are receiving coaching live in the 8-week program on the app or online, we offer recommendations for supplements.

If you experience problems drifting off to sleep regularly, there's a good chance you've already tried some common over-the-counter remedies, including melatonin. But before you pop that pill again, you'll want to read this section thoroughly!

Many people are surprised to learn that I'm not a huge advocate of supplementing with melatonin. While this naturally occurring hormone is vital for establishing good sleep patterns, its use as a sleep aid is not the panacea many believe it is.

Simply put, I don't use melatonin in my brainSHIFT Protocol because it does not resolve the root cause of insomnia.

There is no shortage of sleep supplements to try, and they are found everywhere from your local grocery store to your massage therapist's office. I'd like to break down the ingredients and uses of the supplements research has found to be most effective in both restoring your circadian rhythm and improving sleep quickly.

Melatonin

And let's start with melatonin because my viewpoint and research may surprise you. Melatonin is a naturally occurring hormone in your body that plays a role in sleep. The production and release of melatonin in the brain are connected to the time of day, increasing when it's dark and decreasing when it's light. Melatonin production declines with age.

It is also available as a supplement, which I am reluctant to recommend during the brainSHIFT Protocol.

The cause of sleep disturbances and insomnia are not always easy to identify, but it's an important step in resolving issues in the long run. The leading cause of insomnia is disrupting your circadian rhythm.

What factors cause this disruption in our day-to-day lives? Here are the most common culprits:

• Traveling across time zones

• Working irregular shifts

• Hormone imbalances, alcohol use, and blood sugar levels

• High stress levels or burnout

These root causes need to be identified and addressed for insomnia to improve. Throwing melatonin at the problem ain't gonna fix it.

There are three primary reasons I don't routinely recommend melatonin:

1. In addition to masking or ignoring the root causes of sleep issues, regular use of melatonin can negatively impact hormone levels, particularly when it comes to estrogen and growth hormone.

2. Melatonin also won't help you get back to sleep if you find yourself awake in the middle of the night. You need a more holistic approach to solve this issue.

3. And to make matters worse, using over-the-counter melatonin regularly can actually reduce your ability to produce melatonin naturally.

The fact that melatonin could make your sleep worse and mask bigger issues should give everyone pause.

I'm not completely against the use of melatonin. In fact, it can serve an important role in establishing good sleep patterns—*in specific cases*. But I won't recommend it until all factors have been considered.

As a neurologist, I like to see the results of a sleep study before I recommend a solution. If there is an REM cycle disorder, I might suggest trying out melatonin to see if this helps.

Melatonin can also be beneficial when traveling across multiple time zones. When I'm on a speaking tour, I may use melatonin to get a good night's sleep and combat jet lag. The same goes for shift workers, who may benefit from using melatonin to adjust their circadian rhythm when it's disturbed by shift changes.

When produced by the body, melatonin can help us shift into a bedtime mindset and drift off to sleep more easily. The trick is doing the right things to support our brains to establish healthy circadian rhythms. We will be doing the sleep hygiene routines to reset your circadian rhythm this week as a part of your 7-day sleep challenge.

In some Busy Brain cases, we find melatonin beneficial. Melatonin works best when started at a dose, believe it or not, of 3 mg. I mention that because most of the over-the-counter melatonin you find is a fraction of that dose.

So, be mindful that when you're looking online or in the supplement store, you want a dose of at least 3 mg for adults.

Melatonin has been found in studies to be effective in the following situations:

- Resetting the biological clock to fall asleep earlier in the evening

- Helping prevent symptoms of jet lag

- Helping with middle-of-the-night awakening

Where melatonin does NOT typically help is when it is used as a medication to fall asleep like a sedative. While some people benefit from sedation's side effects, this is not the common use of melatonin.

Magnesium

Research has found magnesium deficiencies in approximately 50% of people in the United States, and the mineral is not easily replaced by nutrition alone. Increased levels of magnesium in the brain have been shown to promote brain function to enhance different forms of learning and memory. In addition, magnesium glycinate has been shown as effective in the treatment of anxiety and insomnia.

When you've been sweating, are dehydrated, or have any alcohol in the evening, your magnesium levels are getting depleted.

A magnesium deficiency negatively affects chemical reactions critical for your brain to sleep (and function). Low magnesium levels will drop serotonin and melatonin levels.

Forms of magnesium I recommend:

1. Magnesium glycinate is the gentlest formulation to avoid stomach upset. Please take this in the evening before

bedtime because it causes sedation and relaxation. Start at 125 mg at night.

2. Magnesium citrate: this version is recommended for constipation, gas, or bloating. It will help both sleep and regular digestion patterns.

One supplement that's used to help boost magnesium levels in those with a deficiency is magnesium glycinate. It's usually well-tolerated and easily absorbed by your body. Magnesium glycinate is the ideal formulation of magnesium. Glycine is an essential amino acid that has important neurotransmitter functions in the brain. Glycine supplementation can improve the quality of sleep, making this form of magnesium a good choice for those with insomnia.

5-Hydroxytryptophan (5-HTP)

5-HTP is a chemical by-product of the protein building block L-tryptophan. It is produced commercially from the seeds of an African plant known as *Griffonia simplicifolia*. 5-HTP works in the brain and central nervous system by increasing the production of the chemical serotonin. Serotonin can affect sleep, appetite, temperature, sexual behavior, and pain sensation.

I often prescribe 5-HTP to clients in low doses, especially if they have a Busy Brain symptom of racing thoughts at night and difficulty staying asleep.

5-HTP is a natural precursor for serotonin, which is also known as the "feel-good hormone" in your brain. The dose we recommend for 5-HTP is to start with 50 mg at night. You can then increase the dose up to 100 mg at night. 5-HTP

can help you fall asleep and stay asleep. This drug is contraindicated and should NOT be taken if you're on an SSRI
or serotonin and norepinephrine reuptake inhibitor (SNRI)
antidepressant medication. Common side effects of 5-HTP
include symptoms like stomach pain, heartburn, nausea, vomiting, and diarrhea. Less commonly, this supplement can cause
adverse effects like headache, insomnia, muscle problems,
and a rapid or irregular heartbeat. Taking very large doses of
5-HTP (more than 600 mg daily) can cause severe muscle
spasms and stomach issues.

And always, please consult your physician and talk to them
before taking any of these supplements.

brainWORK Week 2

The goal of this week's brainSHIFT is to restore your
circadian rhythm, specifically around your sleep-wake
cycle. Some of these steps may seem basic or may be ones
that you have already tried. Don't let the voice of judgment turn you into my Aunties: *Ooooh, I have tried everything to sleep, but I'll only sleep when I stop worrying about
whether Romie will ever find a husband and get married, again.*

The voice of worry is your Busy Brain keeping you
stuck from forward progress. When one worry is re-
solved, another one will replace it to hijack your mind
at night as you try to sleep. You committed to brain-
SHIFT, so let's get started.

brainWORK Step 1

- Set a regular time to go to bed.

- Set a regular time to wake up every morning.

- Keep to the schedule you set regardless of whether you have to work or go to school the next day or it is a day off.

- Try not to worry initially about how many hours of sleep you achieve each night; we want to focus on cultivating a schedule for your brain.

brainWORK Step 2

- Start the 7-day sleep challenge yourself or ask someone you care about to join you. This is also a great team-building exercise at work.

- As our free gift to you, you can download a shareable PDF at *www.BusyBrainCure.com* that goes over how to score your sleep challenge.

- Steps in the sleep challenge also include the following:

  ◊ Clean out the area underneath your bed. Store nothing under your bed. If you have a bed with built-in drawers, no problem. It is time to declutter and organize those drawers.

◊ Remove your work desk from your bedroom.

◊ Remove the television from your bedroom.

◊ Make your bed every morning.

◊ Wash your sheets and place clean sheets on your bed.

◊ Buy an alarm clock for your bedroom to replace your telephone.

◊ Declutter and organize your bedroom closet.

brainWORK Step 3

• Figure out your Busy Brain sleep disturbance pattern.

◊ Pattern I: you have racing thoughts at night that prevent you from falling asleep.

◊ Pattern II: you wake up in the middle of the night and can't fall back asleep.

◊ Pattern III: regardless of how well you slept, you wake up feeling absolutely exhausted and fatigued.

If you have a high Busy Brain score above 30, it is normal to have more than one disturbance or a unique combination of the three I mention above.

If you have more than one Busy Brain sleep disturbance type, start with the lowest number above. So, for example, if you have both sleep pattern types I and III, start with the instructions for sleep pattern type I.

Additional brainWORK Instructions for the 7-Day Sleep Challenge

Use the following checklist to help keep your weekly score.

25 points:

_____ Every night you go to sleep at your scheduled bedtime for up to 7 nights.

_____ Every morning you wake up at your scheduled time for up to 7 mornings.

_____ No work- or school-related activities 30 minutes before bedtime.

_____ Put clean sheets on your bed.

_____ Make your bed every morning.

50 points:

_____ Buy a traditional alarm clock to replace your smartphone.

_____ Declutter and remove anything from underneath your bed.

100 points:

_____ Remove anything work- or school-related from your bedroom, including a computer or desk.

_____ Remove the television from your bedroom.

_____ Clean out and organize your bedroom closet.

Additional brainWORK Instructions for Busy Brain Sleep Pattern Types I, II, III

brainWORK for Busy Brain Sleep Disturbance Type I

To minimize or shut down your racing thoughts at night, try a brainDUMP.

Instructions for a brainDUMP

1. Get a good old-fashioned piece of paper. (No fancy journal required.)

2. Use a pen or pencil and scribble out your work to-do list.

3. Add your home to-do list.

4. Anyone you need to call, email, or text? Write that down too.

5. Random items you meant to google? Record it. You

get the idea. Keep writing in lists. No full sentences are required. Busy Brains often don't have the time or patience to journal regularly.

6. Now pick one thing to prioritize for tomorrow and circle it.

Supplements we recommend, but please first talk to your healthcare provider:

- For 5-HTP, start at 50 mg at night and then increase to 100 mg at night in 7 days if needed.

- Start magnesium glycinate 125 to 200 mg at night.

brainWORK for Busy Brain Sleep Disturbance Type II

To avoid waking in the middle of the night and not being able to go back to sleep:

- Limit caffeine to before noon.

- Consider cutting alcohol consumption by half or stop drinking altogether for just the 7 days.

Supplements we recommend, but please first talk to your healthcare provider:

- 5-HTP 100 mg at night.

- Add magnesium glycinate 125 to 200 mg at night.

brainWORK for Busy Brain Sleep Disturbance Type III

You wake up completely exhausted regardless of how many hours you slept last night. Set your time to sleep at night and wake up every morning, and allow yourself the gift of sleeping an extra 2 to 3 hours if needed. Whatever the root cause of your neuroinflammation, it requires extra time for your Busy Brain's circadian rhythm to restore. In addition, you may need extra sleep as your body and brain are having symptoms of burnout and need the extra rest.

We will discuss the supplements we recommend in the following chapters and at *www.BusyBrainCure.com*. Before you start any supplement regimen, please first talk to your healthcare provider.

We will cover energy boosts in week 5; however, right now, start with a liquid vitamin B complex every morning.

brainWORK for Busy Brain Sleep Disturbance Combination

Again, I wanted to restate that if you have more than one active brain sleep disturbance type, start with the lowest number above. So, for example, if you have both type I and II, start with the instructions for type I.

quickSHIFT: Take Fast Action Now

A reminder: the key this week is to schedule the same time to go to bed and wake up every morning.

Did you know that the most productive people in 2020 and 2021 had one microhabit in common? They got up at the same time every morning.

Bonus quickSHIFT

Really take a peek under your bed and clear out everything.

12

brainSHIFT Protocol, Week 3
Digital Detox

Nancy, a native of the island of Oahu, lost her aloha spirit to video games. When we started the Project Evo research study at Evolution Hospitality, she explained to me that her day working in the hotel was full of encounters—some pleasant but mostly not so pleasant. So, she played video games to numb her mind from work. She woke up early at 4:30 a.m. just to drink coffee and squeeze in gaming for an hour. After work, she counted the minutes until her elderly mother fell asleep so she could compete in the games with strangers for another hour.

When she signed up for the program, she said, "My world recently turned upside down in signing up for the digital detox program. You asked me to give up the only thing I was attached to, and it was hard. But in 4 days, I slept through the night, and people at work told me I looked rested for once.

I decided to continue the program here at Evo for the whole 21 days because it was either detox or Botox for sleep lines."

Within another week, her loved ones came to her perplexed. "Nancy, are you sick and dying? You tell us you love us every day." In addition to her 87-year-old mother, she was a caregiver to her nephew, who was now 12. After giving up video games, online shopping, her iPad, television, and two laptops, she had only one thing left—love. She told everyone in her life that she loved them, daily, including her three rescue dogs, Dottie, Nala, and Max. She was also calling her sister in Seattle, professing her love, and had started weekly family dinners. She closed out one of those Saturday night dinners by giving her iPad to her mom, mailing her laptop to her sister, and giving her Xbox and Wii to her nephew.

"I thought I was only going to do this for 1 month so you could collect data from our company and for your book." But by the end of the 3 weeks, she had not only given away all of her technology devices to other family members but had also stopped drinking alcohol and coffee. "I treated myself to fancy Papyrus paper and a new Montblanc pen, and started to write the poetry that I thought disappeared in me 10 years ago."

Nancy not only reconnected to aloha within her and all around us, she asked me to pass this on to anyone else who was skeptical of starting the program: "I have lived my life asking myself every day if what I am doing is making a difference and what impact it has. I always need to know the impact, good or bad. The impact your program has had is so life-changing to me, and for that, I am so very grateful. Please, please know that it can be life-changing for those that are willing to try."

On behalf of Nancy and her family, aloha and welcome to week 3 of the brainSHIFT Protocol. I'm sure you have already ascertained that this week is about a digital detox for your brain that will improve both your sleep and daytime energy. No need to run to the juice bar or panic about buying some chalky protein shake cleanse system. A cleanse on the brain-SHIFT Protocol does not involve a diet. Remember, comfort food is allowed on the brainSHIFT Protocol. Our goal is to reduce stress levels so you stop stress eating.

In today's world, our lives are surrounded by touch screens, mobile devices, and the normalcy of having multiple screens open on your desktop or multiple screens going in your living room. Research shows that we check our emails an average of seventy-four times a day.

Pause and think about your workspace for a moment. How many screens do you have in use at one time, while having at least one phone to add to the distractions? Can we watch television without simultaneously scrolling social media or googling random facts that are produced by our Busy Brains?

This is me as I wrote the first version of this chapter: "Stop everything. Urgent! Must research what year the brain on drugs commercial came out. Squirrel! Watches *In Living Color* parody involving Kim Wayans's playing Oprah Winfrey repeatedly." I lost forty-two minutes on Wikipedia and YouTube all in the name of "research," which literally was a distraction (albeit one that had me laughing). If you need a dopamine hit from laughter, I have curated a YouTube list of the original commercial, parodies of the campaign, and even a TED talk about the campaign. (Go to *www.BusyBrainCure.com* for a list of the references of random '80s throwbacks I mention in this book.)

brainSHIFT: Digital Detox

Your brain on digital drugs.

If you received a high score on your Busy Brain Test, there's a good chance that you're suffering from stress-induced habits, such as an addiction to the 24/7 news cycle. When Busy Brain symptoms of ruminating anxiety and difficulty paying attention are coupled with sleep deprivation, every news headline feels like a direct threat to your brain. Doomscrolling and doomsurfing have the same effect on your brain as taking a hit of crack or another shot of tequila.

Now a part of the Merriam-Webster dictionary, *doomscrolling* and *doomsurfing* are new terms referring to the tendency to continue to surf or scroll through bad news on TV or online, even though that news is saddening, disheartening, or depressing. Many people are finding themselves continuously reading bad news about current world events without the ability to stop or step back.

Collective eye roll, because I'm right there with you. If you've heard me speak for your company before, your Busy Brain already knows what is coming next, and maybe it will tempt you to shift to the next chapter and skip this one altogether. Before you do, know that in this next step of divorcing digital devices, we are going to work on easy to implement solutions this week, with a few added bonus quickSHIFT ideas once you realize how quickly your Busy Brain can adapt.

So if you have been skimming the last section of this book trying to cherry-pick just a couple of things you can try that feel easy, that is your Busy Brain playing tricks on you. "I already knew this. Why do I need to brainSHIFT?" I know you are looking for the one out of eight brainSHIFTs you are already doing for validation, so you can put the book down and tweet at me, "Hey, Dr. Romie, I've already mastered brainSHIFT. I still have a Busy Brain. Now what?" To that I am going to answer, "Go back to chapter 10. Do each brain-SHIFT 1 week at a time. Don't ignore the hard shit. That's your Busy Brain trying to avoid me."

This is also a gentle but blunt reminder to go back to the previous chapter and start the 7-day sleep challenge. The 7-day sleep challenge is the core principle of resetting our Busy Brains by restoring sleep. But there is one problem for all of us when we try to restore our sleep. Work bleeds into our personal lives; we are expected to check our work emails on our phones at home. Or you may be coming home to spend time with your family and waiting until loved ones go to sleep. You want to cut your quiet time to stay and catch up on work that your Busy Brain distracted you from finishing all day. And I get that that's a reality of all of us success-driven professionals. But you bought this book because a part of you realizes that you need to do something differently. You don't just need random health advice; you are ready to take action.

Stay with me. We are going to do this together. And I really mean it—send me a message on Instagram or LinkedIn that you are committed to week 3 of the brainSHIFT Protocol, and I will cheer you on.

And then do me a favor. Take out your phone as you find my social media accounts on your favorite platform, and set up the do-not-disturb notifications on your phone. Notifications should turn off 30 to 60 minutes prior to you going to sleep.

Yes, we use technology to remind us to detox from digital devices. I am not turning into my Aunties, trying to bring the shiny gold rotary phones back to your home (or mine). And I'm definitely not trying to bring back The Clapper.

Digital Devices and Your Dopamine Reward System

In chapter 9 of section two, you read the inspiring story of Evolution Hospitality's commitment to the well-being of their associates, and the results of how Project Evo changed the way leadership viewed digital devices at bedtime—including Nancy.

I also covered how digital devices reduce our attention span, resulting in adult-onset attention deficit disorder—one of the symptoms of Busy Brain. By the time we get to the brainSHIFTs in weeks 4 and 5, you'll find your focus again by improving your attention span. Using digital devices throughout the day raises dopamine and cortisol levels—thus fueling attention challenges. As we use our digital devices and are exposed to the blue light later into the day and evening, the circadian rhythm of the brain is disrupted. We can no longer experience restorative sleep at night, or have energy during the daytime. Our digital devices, whether it's smartphones, a tablet, laptop computers, gaming devices, or those smart TVs, emit blue light. That blue light goes to the back of your eye on your retina, which goes directly to the airport traffic control center of your brain and says, "Hey, wake up, start stressing and obsessing again." In this week's brainSHIFT, we are going to take steps to start restoring your circadian rhythm and maybe even the love for the people in your household.

Before we get too deep into this week's brainSHIFT, I want to address a question I'm invariably asked at every lecture.

What about the special blue-light-blocking eyeglasses or the filters you can put on the device? Will they alleviate the problem of blue light disturbing your brain's circadian rhythm?

The answer from medical research is no, though it may reduce your eyestrain. Despite wearing blue-light-blocking glasses, exposure to screens will continue to elevate your stress hormones. We have seen in Dr. Yvan Touitou's 2017 published research that when people are looking at a blue light 30 to 60 minutes before bed, their stress hormones cortisol and dopamine rise. But even worse, multiple medical research articles have proven that digital device use before bed will make your feel-good and sleep-good hormones, serotonin and melatonin, totally plummet. So now you're all hyper and stressed out, and the hormones that you need to feel calm and stay asleep and have a happy mood are obliterated. How? All because our Busy Brains led us astray with the toxic habits of doomscrolling. "Oh, let me just scroll down Instagram to unwind, or knock out a few work emails to try to relax before I go to bed." At night, when we're supposed to be trying to calm down, our stress hormone levels go back up with that blue light. Enter your Busy Brain and the racing thoughts we cannot shut down before bedtime.

This week, we are going to start with a digital detox. I welcome you to decide to divorce your digital devices JUST before bedtime. For 7 days. Easy, right? I'm not asking you to divorce them forever or to flush them down the toilet. I want you to know, up front, that I understand we are all living in this hyperconnected society where there are pressures to get work done at home and answer emails or be on social media. But all I'm asking is that for 30 to 60 minutes before bed, you turn off all your devices in your home. Simply start with yourself, but if you do share a bedroom with a partner who likes to watch TV, invite them to join you, or sleep in another room (just until you get through this sleep challenge, but I'm secretly hoping they will join you).

Our course participants often want to invite their kids to do this right away as well, but I'm just going to ask you to be the change you want to see in your household and start with digital detox yourself. So, here's how you get started.

Three Steps of Starting Digital Detox at Bedtime

Step 1: As with the 7-day sleep challenge, I want you to pick a time that you're going to go to bed every night and the time that you're going to get up. And I want you to write that down. There's a contract again for you that's now promising you will try the 7-day sleep challenge. You can download a copy for free if you like at *www.BusyBrainCure.com*.

Step 2: The next step is that once you set your bedtime, I want you to start with 30 minutes if digital detox feels difficult. If you are a go-getter, and you're thinking, "I've already been doing this step since I saw your lecture at my company," I want you to increase digital detox time to 60 minutes.

That means no smartphones, no tablets, no e-readers, no laptop computers, and no TV.

Step 3: Find an activity to do other than using your digital devices. I personally like to wash my dishes at night and take my dog for an extra walk. I'm often scraping off burnt egg from the cast-iron skillet. You can do household chores like preparing meals for the next day. Or try knitting, journaling, adult coloring books, or any activity that keeps your hands busy so you don't pick up that phone again and get tempted. In fact, you can look in the free resources at *www.BusyBrainCure.com* for the favorite activities that our Evolution Hospitality leaders tried successfully while doing their digital detoxes.

Step 4: The next step is to take pen and paper and do a brainDUMP.

The brainDUMP is different than journaling. This is a brainDUMP as a list-making task where single words or random phrases are allowed. Full sentences requiring accurate punctuation and grammar are not required. Take a good old-fashioned pen and paper, and start making a list of the following. You can answer one or all of them.

The first three questions are meant to guide your ruminating anxiety thoughts out from a Busy Brain loop in your brain to paper.

The final four questions are to guide you personally into an assessment of yourself as a leader.

1. What is on your to-do list for your personal life?

2. What is on your to-do list for your workday tomorrow?

3. How do you feel right now? Why?

4. Did you have a moment of gratitude with anyone today, and did you express the gratitude to the person?

5. What went well today?

6. What could you have done differently today?

7. What is one thing you will do tomorrow?

brainWORK Week 3

1. Continue your sleep challenge from week 2, where you had a set time to wake and a time to go to bed.

2. Start a digital detox 60 minutes before your bedtime; if this feels extreme, start with 30 minutes.

3. Find other activities that help create a relaxing ritual prior to bedtime.

4. If you have racing thoughts before bedtime, try a brainDUMP.

quickSHIFTs for Digital Detox

1. Avoid using your phone for an alarm clock. If you have easy access to your phone in the morning, you will be tempted to check your social media or calendar. Avoid raising stress hormone levels before you even get both feet out of bed.

2. Make checking your phone intentional, not compulsive. At your workstation, put your phone 6 to 10 feet away so you have to get up from your desk.

3. Opt out of notifications on your phone, especially news alerts. Also opt out of auto-login for your social media accounts. It feels like an unnecessary hassle, but taking the time to sign back in to your social media accounts creates intentionality over mind-numbing scrolling.

4. Replace something else to touch, smell, or see where your phone used to sit on your desk or nightstand. Examples are essential oils, a photograph in a frame, a vase of flowers, or a stress-relieving squeeze toy. When you have the urge for a dopamine hit by touching and looking at a digital screen, engage with the other item instead.

13

brainSHIFT Protocol, Week 4
brainPAUSE

When I first met Lorraine, she was in the lobby of the hotel where she worked, with a coiffed brunette hairstyle and a warm genuine smile that radiated across the room. This type of hospitality isn't learned; it is in her DNA. After a long day of work and travel, her presence felt like I was sinking into a sofa of my favorite Auntie's house and had been offered a cup of hot chocolate. While she had been in sales at Evolution Hospitality for over 14 years, her business and personal relationships in Southern California spanned decades. Of her many accomplishments as an award-winning sales director, she was most valued as a sought-out mentor and the confidant who all associates turned to in order to share their fears and hopes. Never one to ask for help or advice, she was the person who reveled in being a rock for all those around her.

I first met Lorraine in 2015 when I gave a keynote lecture at Evolution Hospitality's leadership conference. Over the years, as my role grew in the organization into that of Chief Wellness Officer, I came to find Lorraine not only a colleague but also a friend and fellow female leader whom I admired. When the global pandemic started and progressed through 2020, hotels were closed or running at low occupancy. The entire sales team at Evolution Hospitality endured a traumatic period of furloughs, and their sales force was reduced by over 70%. The associates like Lorraine who remained behind not only had to part with talented colleagues who were family but then had to struggle to keep sales in hotel rooms. Struggling to close sales deals for hotels was not common in her region of Southern California, which normally was full of both tourists and convention travelers. Lorraine, like all of our leaders, saw her job duties and role expand while taking a pay cut. She did not let the strain of the time take the kindness out of her smile.

In 2021, as we were starting to slowly emerge from the global pandemic, we launched this 8-week brainSHIFT Protocol to the leaders at Evolution Hospitality to help them recover from Busy Brain and burnout. Lorraine was not only the first person to sign up but rallied other sales leaders who also were suffering from a Busy Brain.

Three weeks into the program, Lorraine's name popped into my inbox, and instinctively I knew something was wrong. Her email started full of gratitude, apologies, and then a polite ask for help in a sorry-to-bother-you manner. I knew something had to be really wrong for her to reach out and ask for help.

By the time I got Lorraine on the phone, her mind was hijacked by repeating thoughts that were hard to string together. I didn't recognize this version of Lorraine; I became worried as I listened to her tense voice, repeating the same fears, worries, and problems over and over again. She would pause to offer a faux solution and then start repeating the fears, worries, and problems yet again.

"Dr. Romie, how can I find another job at my age? No one will hire me as is."

"Hospitality is dead, and I don't know how to work for anyone else."

"It's too early for me to take retirement. I'll take an hourly position at Costco. At least I can shop at a discount."

From all of her worries, I was able to dissect one fact. In the region she covered, several of the company's hotels were being sold and thus were no longer under the Evolution Hospitality management umbrella. She was sure her position would be eliminated, and she would be tossed out of the company. I was listening to her play out multiple scenarios in her mind through her worried voice.

Lorraine's mind was churning with negativity and worrying thoughts on a repeat loop, otherwise known as ruminating anxiety. Ruminating anxiety is a key symptom of a Busy Brain. Lorraine's Busy Brain led her down a path where there was no positive outcome or solution to her predicament. She was convinced that after decades of breaking sales records, she was about to be forced into retirement or resigning from the industry altogether. Her Busy Brain had concocted an entire future where she was left unhirable, undesirable, and unretirable. Future-tripping combined with a Busy Brain had led her to fear losing her home, friends, and 35-year marriage.

She went on to coach me on how to coach her: "And, Dr. Romie, don't tell me to stop and breathe or lead me in a meditation. I tried that multiple times already, and it only makes me feel worse. I can't stop my brain from worrying. I am going to take control, so I made up my mind. When my boss calls, I will resign flat out and give her the speech I have prepared."

And then Lorraine ran out of fuel to sputter out anything more. As I stopped to take a collective breath for the both of us, I knew my one focus was to stop her from preemptively quitting her job and starting a new job at Costco. I then had her rehearse her version of her prepared speech to her boss, announcing that she was quitting, while I listened.

Once she spoke, I asked her how she felt in her body. "Tense all over; something is off."

I then asked her to repeat, "Today is not the day I quit; I will stay another day." She listened and immediately said that her shoulders had released from being adjacent to her ears.

I asked her to wake up every day and repeat the same phrase to herself in the mirror. We were only in week 3 of the program. My goal was to get her to remain focused on finishing this 8-week brainSHIFT program, and at that moment taught her how to brainPAUSE to stop ruminating anxiety.

I checked in with her weekly, and to my relief, she did not quit. By the end of the brainSHIFT program, she reported, "I am shocked at how different I feel completing brainSHIFT. I feel back in control, and my scores (Whole Person 360 Evaluation) have all been reduced by half!" The Whole Person 360 Evaluation is taken inside the 8-week brainSHIFT Protocol Course that we deliver to companies and individuals online.

Rumination and worrying are different symptoms, but both are seen in repetitive negative thoughts and can be associated with anxiety. Lorraine's cycle of negative thoughts is known as rumination. Lorraine was ruminating, and upon further one-to-one evaluation, it was clear she met the criteria for ruminating anxiety. Rumination involves repetitive thinking or dwelling on negative feelings and distress and their causes and consequences. The repetitive, negative aspect of rumination can contribute to the development of both depression and generalized anxiety disorder. Rumination can also worsen preexisting mental health conditions. Rumination is a little different than worrying as it is associated with a sense of loss, hopelessness, and failure. We can see from Lorraine's story above that she was sitting with the idea of herself as a failure despite being an award-winning leader. She was feeling a sense of hopelessness about her job prospects and an understandable sensation of loss.

Worrying is a state of mental distress or agitation due to concern about an impending or anticipated event, threat, or danger. In worrying, we can start to calm ourselves down when we create a solution. However, persistent and repetitive worrying can also lead to anxiety. Ruminating anxiety is defined, then, as rumination that has led to symptoms of generalized anxiety disorder.

brainSHIFT Week 4: brainPAUSE

Why would a high-achieving, successful, goal-oriented professional suddenly feel entirely out of control and start thinking about decisions like abruptly leaving their job, walking out of a marriage, or telling off a lifelong friend? In Lorraine's story above, she had been under chronic stress for over a year, and then an additional stressor occurred—several of the hotels she led were being sold out of the company. Her usual stress-coping techniques were not working for her, and the repetitive negative thoughts were fueling ruminating anxiety. Ruminating anxiety led her to believe she would be given a pink slip and left unemployable. In her Busy Brain, the ruminating thoughts were morphing into her reality. When I was talking to Lorraine, she could already visualize handing out samples as a Costco employee.

Have you ever been in a similar position? I can relate to her situation from my early days of clinical medicine, which you read about in the beginning of this book. Today as I speak and consult, I hear similar stories from high-functioning executives, athletes, lawyers, and doctors alike. Ruminating anxiety is more common in highly intelligent individuals who are used to rationalizing, thinking, and analyzing in their day-to-day professional lives. When we have a Busy Brain, our usual analytical skills turn into anxious analysis or analysis paralysis, and the ruminating anxiety flourishes. When we cannot shut down our ruminating anxiety, it fuels challenges in focusing and completing tasks during the day and falling asleep at night.

As additional stressors get added to our daily schedules, we continue to feel out of control, anxiety worsens, sleep is disrupted, and we are back in the Busy Brain cycle. If you have been stacking the last 2 weeks of brainSHIFTs, we have set a foundation to break the cycle.

And I hear you. The last thing you want me to say is, "Just eat berries and breathe. Everything is going to be all right."

You already have slapped the smartwatch on your wrist that reminded you to stand up or take a mindful minute. Or you have four different meditation apps on your smartphone but are stuck in anxious analysis, wondering which one to open and how to choose from the hundreds of options, and then finding the selection they picked for you annoying.

I wanted to help you train your brain, body, and team this week to learn to take a brainPAUSE. What is a brainPAUSE? I created the term to help all the Busy Brain adults I meet who are in the middle of feeling anxious or suffering from anxiety and are struggling to meditate and quiet their minds.

You are not alone; it is a well-documented scientific phenomenon that when we tell someone who is worrying, ruminating, or has progressed to ruminating anxiety to "calm down, relax, and breathe," it will worsen symptoms.

Steps to Take for a brainPAUSE

Step 1: Step away from the scene of the crime. Our Busy Brains react to what we see, hear, touch, taste, and smell. Our five senses are heightened during periods of stress, sending input to our brain to either continue Busy Brain mode or start to calm down. If a work issue is causing ruminating anxiety, the crime scene is your desk, office, or office building. I want you to imagine a yellow crime tape that you see during a police investigation at a crime scene. Draw a boundary with your imaginary yellow crime tape around your desk, office, or scene of the crime for your Busy Brain. Then walk away. Literally, that may mean excusing yourself to go to the restroom or walking outside the building. The longer you can step away, the easier it is to reset. Being outdoors in nature is ideal for your stress hormone levels; however, the reality is that most of us are in jobs that do not allow us to take a leisurely stroll through a forest in the middle of a work crisis.

Step 2: Reset your senses. Now that you have walked away from the crime scene, it is time to refocus as many of your five senses as possible. Often the easiest is to eat your way through a stressful moment. However, most foods we shovel down in stressful periods will spike our blood sugar, only making ruminating anxiety worse. For ruminating anxiety, powerful tools are music in the form of sound healing and physical sensations such as moving your body.

Option 1: Take a brainPAUSE Using Sound Healing

Music has long been known to soothe and heal the negative impacts of stress on the brain and the body. Music therapy is a well-documented modality used to treat anxiety and other diseases. In recent years, specific modalities such as binaural beats music, sound baths, and various genres of music have been studied in anxiety.

The moment you recognize the ruminating anxiety is limiting you, and you have been able to walk away from the crime scene, the next option is to use sound healing. There are several apps and YouTube videos available that play a specific frequency of music to create a relaxed state to calm anxiety and help sleep. The key is to use your headphones, as the music delivers a subtle frequency difference between your two ears. Studies show sitting for 20 minutes, even for one session, can improve symptoms, and regularly doing this for 2 weeks can reduce anxiety symptoms significantly. You can find a recommendation with our favorite apps and videos at *www.BusyBrainCure.com*.

Option 2: Shake It Off, Literally

I didn't inherit my Aunties' dance skills, specifically bhangra dance, which is native to our Punjabi roots. When music comes on and I dare mosey up to the dance floor, I just look like I am shaking offbeat. Will you join me? Whether you are a dancing queen or a wallflower, I invite you to try shaking therapy. It's also known as therapeutic or neurogenic tremoring, a phrase coined by David Berceli, PhD. The approach involves shaking the body to release tension and trauma, helping to regulate the nervous system.

How do you shake it off? Again, first walk away from the scene of the crime. You can do this seated or standing. Start with one part of your body—an arm or leg—and shake it out. Try to start with 10 to 30 seconds. You can continue to focus on one part of your body or use your entire body. Make silly movements and shake each side of your body. You can use just your limbs or get up and shake your entire body. After 30 seconds, check in and see how your body feels.

Step 3: Optional Supplements for Ruminating Anxiety

In brainSHIFT week 2, we already discussed the benefits of 5-HTP and magnesium glycinate. Both of these supplements, even when taken at night, will start to alleviate the symptoms of ruminating anxiety during the daytime. Between a combination of restoring sleep and improving serotonin levels, symptoms will improve.

An additional option in case 5-HTP is contraindicated for you is to try L-theanine.

The amino acid L-theanine is an effective treatment for moderate and severe anxiety and does not cause drowsiness. It does not interfere with antidepressants or other medications that increase serotonin levels.

Green tea has been utilized for centuries in traditional Chinese medicine and contains many bioactive constituents, including the amino acid L-theanine. Now, L-theanine has been extracted from green tea and is widely used to treat anxiety symptoms. The antianxiety effect of L-theanine is achieved through enhanced alpha brain wave activity and increased synthesis of GABA. Increased GABA, in turn, increases brain levels of dopamine and serotonin, resulting in general feelings of calm and well-being. Gamma-aminobutyric acid (GABA) is a neurotransmitter, a chemical messenger in your brain. It slows down your brain by blocking specific signals in your central nervous system (your brain and spinal cord). GABA is known for producing a calming effect.

Start with 50 mg and increase up to 200 mg. You will feel calm 30 minutes after taking the supplement.

There is no risk of developing tolerance or dependence, and there have been no reports of severe adverse side effects or interactions with other natural products or prescription drugs.

brainWORK Week 4

This week's brainSHIFT is introducing the brainPAUSE. Now is when we also introduce the 3/30 method to learn how to hit the pause button on your Busy Brain. The 3/30 method invites you to take 3-minute pauses during the day and 30 minutes before bedtime. We will continue to build on the previous 3 weeks of brainSHIFTs.

Daytime brainPAUSE

Step 1: Schedule a time to pause during critical moments of your workday. Do not wait for your schedule to get out of control; schedule a pause before a conference call, a team meeting, or working on emails. During this time, walk away from the scene of the crime if possible and reset your senses by focusing on two things you can see, hear, touch, taste, and smell.

Step 2: When you start to feel ruminating anxiety at any time during the day, step away from the scene of the crime and use sound healing or the shake it off method. Download an app to play binaural beats music for anxiety for 20 minutes or go to *www.BusyBrainCure.com* to find our free resources for you to take a brainPAUSE.

Step 3: When you are ready to return to your desk, meeting, or home, pick your focus. Literally say out loud, "I am focused. I am going to focus on _____." And then focus on that next task for 3 to 5 minutes.

Evening brainPAUSE

Step 1: Continue setting a regular time for bed and waking up in the morning from week 2 of the brainSHIFT Protocol.

Step 2: Divorce digital devices and continue 30 to 60 minutes of digital detox before bedtime.

Step 3: Add brainPAUSE to your evening bedtime rituals by using sound healing prior to bedtime, but be mindful not to scroll on your phone if you are using this as a source of music or meditation.

At the time of the writing of this book, Lorraine continued to work successfully at Evolution Hospitality. Then, in late 2022, she was offered a promotion into a new organization overseeing national sales in hospitality. It was a decision she consciously made after she chose to brainSHIFT, and she shared, "I can't even imagine that I thought I was going to leave hospitality or sales last year."

brainSHIFTs Weeks 1 through 4 Summary

Remember, brainSHIFTs build upon the last or stack each week. Here is a summary of the microhabits or brainSHIFTs we have started so far:

1. **Week 1 brainSHIFT:** Set a specific goal and outcome you desire for your 8-week brainSHIFT journey. As we

reach week 4, we are in the middle of the brainSHIFT Protocol. This is a great time to reflect on how far you have come. For example, is your sleep improving in duration and quality? Have you been crossing more tasks off your to-do list?

2. **Week 2 brainSHIFT:** Set a regular time to sleep at night and wake up each morning.

3. **Week 3 brainSHIFT:** It's time to add digital detox 30 to 60 minutes before bedtime. Find other calming rituals to replace screen time before sleep.

4. **Week 4 brainSHIFT:** Schedule a brainPAUSE for 3 minutes during the day and before bedtime.

14

brainSHIFT Protocol, Week 5
Biohack Your Nutrition

Muh mitha karo is a Hindi phrase I often heard from my Aunties as a little girl whenever I would start to lose my cool in my doctor-in-training brain.

When I would become bored or frustrated in childhood, I was sent away to read another chapter in the next volume of the encyclopedia to be trained as a "good-girl-who-is-a-future-doctor." I heard the phrase repeated more frequently as a young woman in medical school when I would give blunt directions to my family that only belonged at work in the hospital wards instead of a loving home.

"Hai, hai, *muh mitha karo*, you cannot talk this bluntly one day to your mother-in-law." (Lord knows I did, which is one of the many reasons I am now divorced. Sorry, not sorry, Aunties.) I was then given a cup of chai and invited to sit with the adults to learn more about the manners of a future bride-to-be.

In my adult life, when this "good girl" became anxious and lost focus as a practicing physician, the overwhelm would cause me to lose my self-control and my calm. The agitating shrill of the pager would refocus my attention to go see the next patient, but I would still be in my Busy Brain. In both instances, loving maternal figures (my Aunties in childhood or the charge nurse in the hospital unit) would sense my need for a reward and fuel me with my only vice—chocolate. I knew I had really made someone mad when they handed me a piece of candy that was out of date and left over from last year's Halloween. I would eat it anyway.

Muh mitha karo literally translates to *sweeten your mouth*. While the goal of this wisdom was to learn to replace my bluntness with politeness and diplomacy, it trained my brain to literally crave sweets—especially chocolate. *Muh mitha karo* is also part of a tradition in our culture to serve sweet food after a spicy meal or difficult task.

Now, as I joyfully polish off a second box of gluten-free Girl Scout cookies in writing the final version of this book, I realize that *muh mitha karo* is the sweet reward in life. Whether from kind and compassionate words or a favorite comfort food, don't we all need more sweetness in our lives?

My ancestry is rooted in the South Asian subcontinent and Ayurveda. Ayurveda is the most ancient form of medicine in the world, dating back over 5,000 years. Today the fancy remedies that line the shelves of natural food stores, like ginger tea, bone broth, and oil pulling, are all based on the rituals of our people.

Ayurveda is a system of medicine based on the idea that an imbalance or stress causes disease in a person's consciousness. In Ayurveda, treatment is based on bringing the whole person—the mind, body, and spirit—back into balance. Interestingly, Ayurvedic medicine has a principle that the body cannot function deprived entirely of sweets. This does not mean eating chocolate, cookies, or cheesecake before the meal. However, we now know that sweets (carbohydrates) are essential for tissue development and restoration and are considered medicinal when consumed in moderation. In traditional Indian cooking, high glycemic white sugar or white flour is rarely used. Eating carbohydrates meant the satiating basmati rice, roti and naan bread, and potatoes.

So my Aunties were proper in their wisdom once again; food is medicine for the spirit. Today, you hear me say food is a love language. So why would we deprive our soul or share the love by forcing diet ideology on one another?

Now, don't mistake my instructions. This is not a hall pass for you to run amok with processed sugars, packaged foods, and french fries in the drive-through of a fast-food restaurant. We discussed the difference between comfort foods and stress eating in section two, chapter 7.

brainSHIFT: Carbs Are Not the Enemy; Make Them Your Ally

Comfort foods are the universal love language that tie us to our families, ancestors, religious or national holidays, countries/regions of origin, and memories. The thread is joy, bliss, and love. During the pandemic, I learned to cook my beloved maternal grandmother's lamb biryani recipe. When I finally got it close, two battling demons were in my Busy

Brain. One was judgment: *Girl, please, you are a hypocrite—there ain't a single anti-inflammatory ingredient in this recipe.* The other voice was of Divine love, feeling like my Nanni was looking over me from above—sending a blessing that I am not alone. Eating that biryani filled me with the inspiration to rebuild my business and do the research you are reading now in this book. Do not let Busy Brain win by shaming you into another cleanse, diet fad, or just following the system your bestie used.

Instead, honor your mind, body, and spirit. By this midpoint in the protocol, the intention is that you are now experiencing restorative sleep. With your circadian rhythm starting to be rebalanced, leptin and ghrelin begin to balance. These are two of many hormones that control your appetite. Leptin decreases your appetite, while ghrelin increases it. Stress eating occurs when cortisol is elevated, thus dropping your blood sugar or affecting mineral balance in the blood and leading to cravings for sugars, carbohydrates, and salty foods in excess. When stress increases, so does ghrelin—and suddenly, you don't understand how you pounded back that stale bag of nacho cheese Doritos from the back of your pantry when you haven't touched the stuff in years.

I am not shaming anyone who has found a nutrition plan that works for them and can maintain the strict rituals. However, have you failed any of the latest fad diets? In my extensive research to find the right nutrition plan, there is no doubt eating low glycemic foods and anti-inflammatory foods promotes brain and gut health.

Have you tried eating clean before? How long did it last before you "cheated"? In my integrative medicine practice, I had a roster full of clean eaters rigid on their vegan, Whole30, paleo, Atkins, or ketogenic diets. And they still suffered from Busy Brains.

It was, however, in being on the ground as a Chief Wellness Officer for over 7,000 employees that the reality of the situation became clear. Life is complicated and full of daily stressors, and in addition, I served a diverse workforce. Most of us spend energy trying to balance work and a semblance of a personal life. The top ten trendy diet plans tell me that the American wellness market does not account for the cultural foods of most of the world's religions, countries, races, and ethnicities.

In brainSHIFT, the goal is that everyone has a seat at the table, whether you are a vegan, chocolate lover, paleo, or confused about what to eat and making a run for the coffee shop.

Caffeine-Carb Rule of Thumb

Do you add sugar when you go to your local coffee shop or take afternoon tea? Or, after a meal that includes rice, pasta, or potatoes, do you now need coffee to return to work? Whether you add sugar to your caffeinated beverage or eat high glycemic foods with your meal, combining sugar and caffeine will worsen your Busy Brain symptoms. I reflect on my days as an attending physician fueled on coffee to work through 12- to 14-hour days. Adding chocolate or any sweet rewards would give me a few seconds of an energy buzz, but ultimately I would get even more frazzled, anxious, and behind in my work after I crashed from that high. Does that happen to you as well during your workday? High glycemic carbohydrates primarily determine this energy roller coaster.

As a reminder from section two, chapter 7 of the book, we define high glycemic foods as carbohydrates that are quickly digested and absorbed, causing a rapid rise in blood sugar. Examples of high glycemic foods are white sugar, white flour, white rice, white potatoes, and white bread. My Indian Aunties may have something to say about all the whiteness here—but I'll be polite. "Aunties, *muh mitha karo*—remember?"

This week's brainSHIFT is designed to help you choose one: either consume caffeine or high glycemic foods, but avoid combining both of them in one meal or snack. If you consume high glycemic foods, you must avoid caffeine for at least 1 hour before and 1 hour after. This brainSHIFT also means no adding sugar to your tea, coffee, or soda. If you are in the mood for *muh mitha karo* after a spicy meal or stressful moment in your day, then skip the caffeinated beverage.

My Aunties are doing a facepalm here. "Hai hai, what am I going to serve when company comes over for chai in the afternoon? I just ordered the fancy tea biscuits from Harrods. What about after serving spicy haleem and biryani for dinner? No good hostess would refuse, *muh mitha karo*. Dessert after a heavy, spicy meal is a basic hosting duty."

Whether it's cookies with afternoon tea, bagels with morning iced coffee, or a croissant with an espresso, so many of us have the habit of quickly grabbing what feels like a one-two punch of energy for our brain. Sugar followed by caffeine. What I'm asking you to do is to pick one or the other, but not both at the same time.

The truth is that sugar in your brain promotes inflammation that will depress serotonin levels—and we worked so hard in the first 4 weeks of brainSHIFT to restore your serotonin levels to help sleep and sanity. I don't want to deprive you of carbohydrates, just minimize the effects on Busy Brain.

When we combine caffeine and white sugar, we overload the Busy Brain circuits, worsening anxiety and attention deficit. The result? You'll feel more anxious and self-critical over the to-do list that has not been tackled but only multiplied in its length and intensity. So conversely, if you drink a caffeinated beverage, make sure you avoid sugar, white sugar, raw sugar, honey, agave syrup, white flour, white rice, white potatoes, and white bread. You get the idea.

Let me be clear: I am not against sugar/high glycemic index foods. I want to give you the most powerful microhabit or brainSHIFT to help you calm your Busy Brain. After decades as a practicing physician in neurology and integrative medicine, I know that staying on a low glycemic index diet permanently is challenging if not near impossible. My Aunties are not the only ones who live by *muh mitha karo*. The most powerful action you can take to brainSHIFT is to pick one or the other.

Is a nutrition plan really this simple? In late 2022, we ran the brainSHIFT 8-week course for a group of educators. Felicia is a school principal for a large district in the state of New York and joined the program stating that her sleep was not only good but lasted 8 to 9 hours. She would wake up without wanting to eat breakfast, but by midmorning, she would crash. Felicia stuffed packets of instant oatmeal in her work bag for snacks and yet found that her energy continued to feel drained all day. By the time she started brainSHIFT, she was questioning whether she was too old (in her early 50s) to handle the job's demands. She followed this one brainSHIFT and switched the high glycemic instant oatmeal for overnight oats. She added berries and ate that midmorning. She waited until she arrived at the school to drink coffee and replaced honey with stevia. Within 1 week, she said she was energized, needed less caffeine, and was refocused.

brainWORK Week 5

Congratulations, you've made it to the halfway point in the brainSHIFT Protocol. In the first 4 weeks, we spent time stacking microhabits (brainSHIFTs) to restore sanity and sleep. Weeks 5 to 8 focus on what I call your energy blueprint. We are now going to brainSHIFT to boost your daytime energy, focus, and mood.

This week, we're going to talk about getting explicitly focused on how you fuel yourself and what foods you're using.

This week, the brainSHIFT is a quick biohack for your nutrition:

1. If you consume a beverage or food with caffeine, please avoid these five foods within 1 hour of your caffeine: white sugar, white rice, white potatoes, white bread, and white flour.

2. To sweeten your caffeinated beverage, use a low glycemic sweetener like stevia or coconut oil.

3. Try to substitute low glycemic foods into each of your

meals. If that feels overwhelming, start with just one meal. Examples of these low glycemic foods are sweet potatoes and quinoa.

Do you want a full list of low glycemic index foods you can continue to eat? In appendix B, we give you a list of low glycemic index foods to fuel your brain and body.

4. I learned that mangos keep our family tradition of *muh mitha karo*.

If you do this one simple hack this week, you'll feel more focused. When we ran the brainSHIFT Protocol for our corporate teams, the first 48 hours felt uncomfortable due to changes in habits and sugar consumption. By the end of the week, individuals reported having more energy and decreased belly bloating.

brainSHIFTs Weeks 1 through 5 Summary

Remember, brainSHIFTs build upon each previous week. Here is a summary of the microhabits or brainSHIFTs we have started so far:

1. **Week 1 brainSHIFT:** Set a specific goal and outcome you desire for your 8-week brainSHIFT journey. As we reach the middle of brainSHIFT, this is a great time to reflect on how far you have come. For example, is your sleep improving in duration and quality? Have you been crossing more tasks off your to-do list?

2. **Week 2 brainSHIFT:** Set a regular time to sleep at night and wake up each morning.

3. **Week 3 brainSHIFT:** It's time to add digital detox 30 to 60 minutes before bedtime. Find other calming rituals to replace screen time before sleep.

4. **Week 4 brainSHIFT:** Schedule a brainPAUSE for 3 minutes during the day and before bedtime.

5. **Week 5 brainSHIFT:** This week, you are avoiding high glycemic foods (white sugar, white flour, white potatoes, white rice, and white bread) within 1 hour of consuming caffeine.

quickSHIFT: Take Fast Action Now

Want to help prolong the brain-boosting effects of your coffee?

We borrow from the traditions of *po cha* traditional Tibetan butter coffee. Typically, *po cha* is made with fermented yak butter and black tea. A natural and healthy fat is combined with caffeine to prolong the brain-boosting effects.

In the West, companies like Bulletproof coffee have created similar recipes using low-mold organic coffee and their signature oils that contain medium-chain fatty acids (healthy fats).

In brainSHIFT, we recommend the following recipe of ingredients you can find easily at your local supermarket:

1. Brew organic coffee, preferably fair trade beans, ground fresh.

2. Add 1 to 2 tablespoons of organic coconut oil.

3. Add 1 tablespoon of organic unsalted butter.

Note: we have tried the above recipe with tea—and, well, let's say coffee tasted better. I learned not to mess with the traditional chai recipe from my Aunties ever again. You can find these recipes at *www.BusyBrainCure.com.* If you have a tasty alternative recipe to share utilizing tea and medium-chain fatty acids, please send it over to me, and we'll share your idea with the global brainSHIFT community.

15

brainSHIFT Protocol, Week 6
Fuel, Energy, and Focus

"Intermittent fasting is all the rage these days, right? The latest trend? Want to hear my version? I eat my last bit of chocolate around 9:00 p.m., and absolutely no more food after that. Maybe one more Lindt truffle at 9:01 p.m., but then that's it. For real. I wake at 8:00 a.m., and because my menagerie of animals are all vying for my attention, I get up and feed my colony of feral cats in the garage as they climb the legs of my Carhartt overalls. I run in the house and mix up yogurt and pumpkin for my three spoiled-rotten dogs because dogs need their probiotics, too. I do manage to pour myself an iced coffee to take with me as I run to the barn before my horses kick a hole through their stall walls because I haven't thrown them hay yet. Chores take me about 3 hours each morning. So that's 14 hours without food. Voila! Intermittent fasting, farm girl style."

This was Melanie's confession to me as she was editing the

previous chapter of this book when we discussed diet fads and the brainSHIFT of choosing either caffeine or a high glycemic food at each meal. In addition to her love of horses, Melanie works as a developmental editor.

I first met Melanie in 2013 when I was transitioning from traditional neurology into integrative medicine. She was one of the first people who heard about my idea and mission, and instead of judging me, she lovingly encouraged me to follow my path. Since that time, she's served as an unofficial Auntie in my business, always offering laughter, a pragmatic assessment, and loving wisdom when a new idea was taking shape. Melanie was the first person to hear about the concept of this book and helped me map out a plan when I started the research several years prior to starting the writing. When I knew the research on the Busy Brain Cure was ready, she was the Auntie I ran to with my disorganized notes.

Melanie read chapter 1, took the Busy Brain Test, and left a note in the margin. "Yikes, help. I scored an 85 on the test!" I thought it was an 83, but always the overachiever, she wanted the extra two points for emphasis.

"Your book could not have come at a better time. I think I have a Busy Brain, and I'm wondering if Busy Brain could be making my Hashimoto's thyroid disease worse?"

In the several months that went by as I wrote each chapter of this book, we had weekly check-in calls. Each week, Auntie Melanie unwrapped a little bit more information about her complex and lengthy medical history. I learned that Melanie had a myriad of symptoms that were rooted in her Busy Brain and her immune system. She has spent decades under the care of both traditional Western doctors and integrative medicine practitioners, following every plan, diet, and medication regimen as prescribed. She told me about her Busy Brain and how it impacted the life she cultivated for herself and her animals on her farm.

"I worked hard to build a retreat space surrounded by nature for clients to do writing and Equus work. I have a wonderful workload with clients I adore and the peace I find with all my animals: dogs, cats, and horses alike. Yet I find myself experiencing anxiety almost every day. When I'm working, or with my animals, or when I'm out in nature, I feel a full sense of presence and peace, but outside of that, when I'm left with just myself, I feel anxious most of the time. I eat reasonably well, aside from the chocolate/sweets. I exercise robustly every single day, walking 5 miles or more and lifting 80-pound bales of hay, and my body hurts 99% of the time. In those moments, I feel like I'm in a state of flight or fight. Or as if I'm unmoored."

There's something to be said about the stress on the brain that a rigid protocol would bring into her already complex daily schedule managing her chores on her farm, caring for horses, writing her own book, and editing the writing of multiple authors. Her symptoms of difficulty focusing, anxiety, and sleep challenges persisted as we were mapping out the brainSHIFT Protocol.

Initially, she pushed back on sleep issues, and then remembered, "Oh, okay, full disclosure: I was diagnosed with severe sleep apnea in 2017 and had to use a CPAP sleep machine for several years. I've taken a low dose of Ambien each night ever since because that damn machine was horrendously blowing a hard stream of air in my face and it made me feel claustrophobic. But…now I do sleep from when I lie down until morning with a full 8 hours almost every night. But as of 2019, after my last sleep test, I no longer have sleep apnea." I summoned my best *muh mitha karo* attitude and reminded her that it was now 2022 as she told me her sleep history. Perhaps another sleep study would help?

She felt relief when she read in the protocol that her favorite high glycemic foods are allowed—just avoid caffeine. She followed last week's brainSHIFT, and then I added, "Allow yourself the luxury of being a farm Auntie and put two slabs of your farm-fresh butter into your coffee with coconut oil before you go in to care for the horses every morning."

Oops, she didn't tell me it was iced coffee, even on snowy days. Evidently eating frozen chunks of coconut oil creates a chewy coffee experience.

She then was instructed to add one healthy fat to each meal she ate, while following the previous week's brainSHIFT. Melanie said she'd never been eating more foods that are prohibited on all of the trendy nutrition protocols she had been prescribed in the past. I could hear relief each week as we celebrated the comfort foods we ate. Hers were the idyllic recipes and comforts of farm life: made-from-scratch cookies, homemade baked bread, and of course that farm-fresh butter. After 2 weeks of following these brainSHIFTs, it was no surprise to me that Melanie reported, "You mean your program isn't as restrictive as only turkey and vegetables for 6 months—or eating raw amaranth?" Food is the medicine for the spirit.

This week's brainSHIFT is simple and designed to fuel your brain and body through the day: add one healthy fat to every meal.

brainSHIFT

Sticking to any of the rigid diet protocols like Melanie had tried for over a decade, such as one in which she described cutting all food except white turkey breast and a small list of approved vegetables for almost 6 months before she was allowed to begin reintroducing foods such as raw amaranth (which still causes her to shudder), feels like a full-time job and starts to increase stress levels. Instead, I wanted to research the most potent brainSHIFTs to fuel your brain and body while boosting your daytime energy at the same time.

I also wanted you to have the comfort of consuming your favorite foods on a schedule, rather than using food for stress management. Whether it's Melanie's baked-from-scratch sourdough bread slathered in organic butter or me cooking my Nanni's Punjabi biryani recipe, allow the food of your people to offer the healing our Busy Brains need. In appendix C, you will find the comfort foods of the people I love. They are the people who have given me comfort in all the stages of my life, from budding doctor-to-be to the now STEMinist in Stilettos.

How can we accomplish all of this? This week's biohack for your nutrition is simple. Make a list of healthy fats that you enjoy eating that are rich in omega-3 fatty acids and DHA. And then, take one to two servings of these healthy fats and add to every meal.

Foods that are rich in omega-3 fatty acids include:

1. Fish and other seafood (especially cold-water fatty fish, such as salmon, mackerel, tuna, herring, and sardines)

2. Nuts and seeds (such as flaxseed, chia seeds, and walnuts)

3. Plant oils (such as flaxseed oil, soybean oil, and avocado oil)

You can see a full list in appendix B or download the list at *www.BusyBrainCure.com*.

Did your Busy Brain just start to panic? "Yikes, did you say fatty foods?"

As we covered in chapter 8, the root cause of Busy Brain symptoms is a specific pattern of neuroinflammation that disrupts how your brain cells communicate. To calm the inflammation that causes a Busy Brain, healthy fats are a key component of the nutrition required in your brain.

In a standard diet promoting low-fat consumption, fat intake is unbalanced. Low omega-3 polyunsaturated fatty acids (n-3 PUFAs) have been associated with neuropsychiatric and neurological disorders with inflammation, including ruminating anxiety, ADHD, and insomnia. Yes, one of the unwanted side effects of decades of a low-fat diet is symptoms of a Busy Brain. In addition to fueling your brainPOWER, consuming healthy fats will also reduce your harmful belly fat.

Leptin signals your brain that you are full and to stop eating. Leptin also supports efficient metabolism. If too much leptin builds up in your blood, you may develop leptin resistance. When this occurs, the leptin in your body may not do its job effectively, resulting in weight gain. The mechanisms that can cause leptin to build up in your bloodstream? You guessed it—sleep deprivation, stress, and a Busy Brain. Cortisol, one of the hormones that is elevated when you have a Busy Brain, may make your brain less receptive to leptin and cause you to overeat.

The conclusion, if you have a Busy Brain, is that your elevated stress hormones may be blunting your ability to lose weight. Eating healthy fats is one of the key nutrition recommendations for restoring your leptin levels (in addition to sleep). By the end of weeks 5 and 6 of brainSHIFT, 60% of our participants reported reduced belly bloating, a drop in pants/dress size, and losing weight.

brainWORK Week 6

1. Make a list of foods you enjoy that are rich in omega-3 fatty acids.

2. Add at least one serving of healthy fats to every meal and snack you have daily.

3. Fish oil supplements: In clinical studies, effective doses range from 500 to 2,000 mg daily. It is vital to find a supplement where the omega-3 fatty acid ratio is higher than the omega-6 fatty acid ratio. The main omega-3s present in fish oil are eicosapentaenoic acid (EPA) and docosahexaenoic acid (DHA), which impact brain development and function.

brainSHIFTs Weeks 1 through 6 Summary

Remember, brainSHIFTs build upon each previous week. Here is a summary of the microhabits or brainSHIFTs we have started so far:

1. **Week 1 brainSHIFT:** Set a specific goal and outcome you desire for your 8-week brainSHIFT journey.

2. **Week 2 brainSHIFT:** Set a regular time to sleep at night and wake up each morning.

3. **Week 3 brainSHIFT:** It's time to add digital detox 30 to 60 minutes before bedtime. Find other calming rituals to replace screen time before sleep.

4. **Week 4 brainSHIFT:** Schedule a brainPAUSE for 3 minutes during the day and before bedtime.

5. **Week 5 brainSHIFT:** This week, you are avoiding high glycemic foods (white sugar, white flour, white potatoes, white rice, and white bread) within 1 hour of consuming caffeine.

6. **Week 6 brainSHIFT:** This week, you are making a list of healthy fats you enjoy eating and adding one to two servings of healthy fats to each meal.

quickSHIFT: Take Fast Action Now

If you choose fish oil supplements, take these daily at bedtime with vitamin D3 to also assist in the absorption and metabolism of vitamin D3—a preview for next week's brainSHIFT.

16

brainSHIFT Protocol, Week 7
Superbrain Superhormones

I always have a nervous energy when we reach the final week of the program with a company. If I have a Busy Brain moment, fear comes in: *Will anyone show improvement? Will their CEO/VP of human resources/CFO think the investment was worth it?* And then I follow my own advice and take a brainPAUSE. I remind myself that I created this protocol and entire program after repeating these steps for all of my clinic patients I used to see as a neurologist and integrative medicine doctor. I then remind myself what I learned from my mindfulness and spiritual teachers. *Your job is to show up without attachment, listen, encourage, and share compassion.*

In early 2021, one of the first larger teams to start the brainSHIFT 8-week live program was having their virtual finale party, and someone whom I hadn't noticed on any call before raised their hand, and in the Zoom chat asked to be brought onto the screen live, with the company's president. I took another deep, cleansing breath and gave her the stage.

"I started this program skeptical, thinking you were a bit out there, Dr. Romie. I would have never signed up for this alone, let alone followed your instructions to see my doctor. I only showed up because my team here at work was excited to start brainSHIFT," Kelly said to me on video with the president of her company, and over 120 of her colleagues wondering where this story would go next. She jumped right in.

"I was afraid a doctor would judge me, tell me that I am crazy, or even worse, that my nonstop anxious feelings were all in my head, and I didn't want to be put on a medication I could never stop. But when all of my colleagues started making appointments with their doctors to get their labs, I followed suit."

As you have guessed from previous chapters, the brainSHIFT Protocol encourages (but does not force) you to consider getting key labs drawn that require your physician to order and follow up with them. When we deliver the program to any company, the sleep challenge that is completed as a brainSHIFT for week 2 is done as a team competition, often with prizes for whoever did the best. Kelly further went on to tell all of us that she only went along for the sake of winning said prize, and even as she started to add hours of sleep back into her life each night and felt a little better, she couldn't quite put her finger on why. While she played along and added each brainSHIFT every week and felt improvement, there wasn't a complete resolution of her anxiety.

"Until I got my labs back," she added. "Initially, my doctor wasn't sure about running all these labs, but then the shocking news came. My thyroid panel was completely abnormal. My doctor then ordered an ultrasound, found a nodule, and now I will have it biopsied next week."

The fear in her voice was palpable, and I had tears streaming down my face, trying to stifle sobs. *I've been there before, Kelly. I got your back.*

"They started me on medication for my thyroid, and for the first time in years, I feel like I have an answer. My doctor said this program saved my life. Had you not insisted on these labs, it could have been a fatal cancer in my thyroid that was discovered only when it was too late. Bringing brainSHIFT to our company saved my life, Dr. Romie. And I have to admit, it was my Busy Brain and my fear stopping me from admitting to the doctor that I have crippling anxiety and was struggling to focus and cope at work."

I was stunned into silence. What a courageous leader to share her story on a virtual call with camera on in front of the company's president and 120 leaders. As a human resource manager, she was normally on the receiving end of hearing other people's trauma, drama, and life stressors. And here she was, modeling vulnerability and hope.

I still get choked up when I think of these clients who've had such profound results, even though we have breakthroughs like Kelly's in every cycle of brainSHIFT that we run for groups and teams. Every. Damn. Time. And just like Kelly, many leaders torture themselves with their beliefs that their Busy Brain symptoms mean they are somehow inferior to their peers or are not cut out to succeed at their companies in their current roles. A Busy Brain can give anyone a judgmental Auntie talking back to them.

Read this next line out loud. Your Busy Brain is not a product of your imagination, a character flaw, or the drawing of a bad tarot card. The actual root cause of a Busy Brain can be a thyroid hormone disorder, low vitamin D3 levels, insulin resistance, or an autoimmune disorder that has gone undiagnosed, ignored, or untreated. All these are the root causes we discussed in section two of the book (just in case you skipped all the sciency stuff).

brainSHIFT

Kelly is not an isolated case. About 30 to 40% of subclinical hypothyroid and hypothyroid disease cases have an anxiety disorder, difficulty focusing, and sleep disturbance. As I explained in chapter 6, subclinical hypothyroid disease is routinely missed in women because they have symptoms consistent with hypothyroid disease, but lab work shows a "normal" thyroid-stimulating hormone (TSH) level. Subclinical hypothyroid disease is often diagnosed when an expanded lab testing is completed for the thyroid gland. Hypothyroid disease is based on both symptoms and abnormal lab values of the TSH level.

But first, we must get you across the finish line—or even started on the track. This week's brainSHIFT is a request to check your labs from your physician. At the end of this chapter, I list the main labs to screen in the brainWORK section. You'll also find an expanded laboratory evaluation list in appendix A and online at *www.BusyBrainCure.com*.

Why all of these labs? As we discussed in section two of the book, having a Busy Brain is not a character flaw you possess, but often there is an underlying root cause. I have listed the most common causes here and then tips on discussing these issues with your physician.

Getting Down to the Root Cause of Busy Brain

A Busy Brain can develop due to an underlying root cause that may be missed, ignored, or not assessed fully by your primary care physician. This is why I wrote the book. (Give a copy to your doctor. I have had many colleagues as my clients over the years.)

In section two, chapters 6 and 7, I dug deeper into the science and medical research of neuroinflammation related to the Busy Brain. While there are many causes a trained integrative medicine physician can screen for, I wanted to focus on the most common issues that not only clinicians face but that we also see with our participants in the 8-week brain-SHIFT program.

There are four essential regions to look for issues:

1. Methylation disorders

2. Thyroid hormones

3. Blood sugar control

4. Vitamin D3 levels

Before you go googling how to take an online test for symptoms concerning a potential thyroid, blood sugar, or vitamin D3 imbalance you may have, I am here to tell you this. As a physician, the only way to truly ascertain that you have an issue is to have your labs drawn. I know I just made it difficult for you; you actually have to stop skimming these chapters and take action here. Now, this microhabit is not mandatory—but aren't you the slightest bit curious about what is happening with the hormones and chemistries in your body?

Methylation Disorders

You don't need to run and grab a 23andMe kit or start hunting down your ancestry to see if any of your Aunties are responsible for your Busy Brain. I'm not insulting your Aunties; my Aunties would choke on their chai if I disrespected your elders. If one of your Aunties has a methylation disorder, it may run in the family. While many genetic diseases can affect the brain and mental health, the one key genetic disease I screen for is methylation disorders. Under this category, the most common is the methylenetetrahydrofolate reductase (MTHFR) mutation.

The MTHFR enzyme plays an essential role in processing amino acids, specifically converting homocysteine to methionine. Methionine is an essential amino acid that is required to build proteins in the body. MTHFR produces an essential enzyme that converts folate into a form that plays a role in mood-regulating neurotransmitter production. Being diagnosed with the MTHFR mutation is an opportunity to change your diet and lifestyle to maximize your methylation, manage symptoms, and optimize your overall health.

When an MTHFR mutation occurs, there is a risk of elevated markers of neuroinflammation and inflammation in the body. MTHFR deficiency is the most common genetic cause of elevated levels of homocysteine in the plasma (called hyperhomocysteinemia) and reduced levels of folic acid in the blood. While there are many risks associated with MTHFR mutation, from cardiovascular disease to an increased risk of miscarriages, two important medical problems linked to this deficiency are anxiety and attention deficit disorder.

Thyroid Hormone Disorder

For both men and women, the thyroid gland is a key component of all of our metabolic functions for the brain and the body. As discussed in detail in section two, chapter 6, the thyroid gland function is key in maintaining mood, energy, and attention.

Too often, a thyroid disorder is missed because of an incomplete list of symptoms from a patient and/or a lab only checking one laboratory value—the thyroid-stimulating hormone (TSH). This means as a part of a routine screening, a doctor will see that your TSH is within a broad normal range and dismiss symptoms like lack of daytime energy and anxiety.

In our lab panel, we ask that your physician order a full thyroid panel that includes the following laboratory values:

1. Thyroid-stimulating hormone (TSH)

2. Total triiodothyronine T3

3. Total thyroxine T4

4. Free triiodothyronine (fT3)

5. Free thyroxine (fT4)

6. Reverse T3 (rT3)

7. Anti-thyroglobulin antibodies

8. Thyroid peroxidase antibodies

The reason we are screening with all of these labs, as we discussed in chapter 6, is that too often the following root causes of a Busy Brain can be missed:

1. Autoimmune thyroiditis

2. Subclinical hypothyroidism

3. Subclinical hyperthyroidism

Blood Sugar Control (Insulin Resistance)

You may be rolling your eyes now, thinking, "Dr. Auntie Romie, you said I could eat comfort food, and now we are going to bring up blood sugar." Yes. By now, 7 weeks into the brainSHIFT Protocol, the hope is that you have stopped or curbed stress eating by restoring your circadian rhythm in the first 4 weeks and then by creating nutrition biohacks in the last 2 weeks. These brainSHIFTs should have moderated the yo-yo effect of your blood sugar. Our former participants in brainSHIFT found that they craved fewer sweets or high glycemic foods by week 6, and it became easier to choose slow carbs over foods that spiked their blood sugar to give that quick rush and crash.

Remember, eating comfort food is always allowed. How many comfort food meals are you allowed? Schedule your comfort meals once to twice a week that are tied to eating food that is in celebration or honor of life, religion, loved ones, culture, heritage, or ancestry. We are eating mindfully rather than eating to calm stress or a Busy Brain. Typically I see that by the time we reach weeks 5 through 8 of the protocol, stress eating has subsided.

However, without labs, we cannot assume that your symptoms mean that you have insulin resistance. Insulin resistance is when cells in your muscles, fat, and liver don't respond well to insulin and can't easily take up glucose from your blood. Insulin resistance is a pathway to developing metabolic syndrome, increased risk of diabetes mellitus type 2, and other diseases. There are many causes, including stress—as we discussed in chapter 7.

Insulin has two crucial functions in the brain: controlling food intake and regulating cognitive functions, particularly memory. Brain insulin resistance also alters dopamine turnover and induces anxiety and depressive-like behavior. This is especially true in a Busy Brain when the airport traffic control tower has disrupted the hypothalamic–pituitary–adrenal axis (HPA axis), leading to disruption in cortisol, growth hormone, catecholamines, and/or glucagon.

I covered the reasons behind all of these laboratory values in chapters 6 and 7. The laboratory evaluations we seek here are the following:

1. Fasting blood sugar level

2. Hemoglobin A1c (HbA1c)

3. Fasting insulin level

4. Triglycerides and total cholesterol panel

5. Serum sex hormone-binding globulin

Vitamin D3 Levels

We discussed in chapters 6 and 7 that vitamin D should be relabeled as a prohormone or superhero vitamin of your brain and body. It's estimated that 50% of people globally have insufficient levels of vitamin D, which are measured in nanograms per milliliter (ng/mL) clinically or sometimes referred to in nanomoles per liter (nmol/L) in the research literature. In clinical studies, vitamin D, especially vitamin D3, plays a vital role in brain plasticity and neuroimmunomodulation. It is derived from sunshine and fish containing higher fat. Unfortunately, due to inflammation and other causes, even those people living in warm weather climates suffer low vitamin D levels. Research has suggested a relationship between vitamin D deficiency and vulnerability to depression and anxiety as well as a whole host of other neurological and psychiatric symptoms. This is one of the supplements that is likely needed where diet and time in sunshine alone will not resolve the issue. I cover in chapters 6 and 7 the "normal range" that is accepted by traditional medicine. In our fields of integrative and functional medicine, we do not wait for your bones to fracture to assess vitamin D3 levels. Therefore, to keep your health optimized, you will find it's important to optimize your vitamin D3 levels earlier and with more targeted precision.

To properly assess your vitamin D3 levels, we recommend you obtain the following laboratory evaluations:

1. 25-hydroxyvitamin D (25(OH)D)

2. 1,25-dihydroxyvitamin D (1,25(OH)$_2$D)

brainWORK Week 7

So this week, the brainWORK is echoing brainWORK from week 1—to make an appointment with your primary care provider and ask them to order laboratory tests to assess the root cause of your Busy Brain (and/or the long-term complications of a Busy Brain).

You can see the full list of laboratory evaluations for men and women in appendix A, or download your suggested laboratory evaluation at *www.BusyBrainCure.com*.

Here is a pro tip for individuals in the United States in advocating for these labs with your primary care provider.

1. Many of the labs are a part of a routine annual wellness check to screen for diseases or risk factors for developing disease (such as screening cholesterol levels and blood sugar levels).

2. It is important to tell your physician that you want additional labs done due to your symptoms related to a Busy Brain, which may include fatigue, disturbed sleep (insomnia), difficulty focusing, difficulty losing/gaining weight, or anxiety. Insurance will cover many

of the laboratory tests if there is a valid diagnosis or symptom for the reason the labs are being checked. In other words, do not just walk in and say, "Can you check these labs because I am reading a book called *The Busy Brain Cure?*"

3. Having said that, if your primary care provider has more questions, give them a copy of this book. Section two covers all of the science and reasoning. I have additional scientific references for all of the medical journal articles in the bibliography and online at *www.BusyBrainCure.com*.

brainSHIFTs Weeks 1 through 7 Summary

Remember, brainSHIFTs build upon themselves each week. Here is a summary of the microhabits or brainSHIFTs we have started so far:

1. **Week 1 brainSHIFT:** Set a specific goal and outcome you desire for your 8-week brainSHIFT journey.

2. **Week 2 brainSHIFT:** Set a regular time to sleep at night and wake up each morning.

3. **Week 3 brainSHIFT:** It's time to add digital detox 30 to 60 minutes before bedtime. Find other calming rituals to replace screen time before sleep.

4. **Week 4 brainSHIFT:** Schedule a brainPAUSE for 3 minutes during the day and before bedtime.

5. **Week 5 brainSHIFT:** This week, you are avoiding high glycemic foods (white sugar, white flour, white potatoes, white rice, and white bread) within 1 hour of consuming caffeine.

6. **Week 6 brainSHIFT:** This week, you are making a list of healthy fats you enjoy eating and adding one to two servings of healthy fats to each meal.

7. **Week 7 brainSHIFT:** Call your primary care physician's office and make an appointment to have your labs checked, especially if you are still having Busy Brain symptoms after completing weeks 1 through 6. You can find a list of the partial labs in appendix A and a full list on the online program at *www.BusyBrainCure.com* or download the brainSHIFT app.

quickSHIFT: Take Fast Action Now

At the writing of this book, the number of online medical companies has expanded in the United States where you can pay to have your labs drawn, and these facilities are supervised by a licensed physician. These companies may or may not accept traditional health insurance or payments from your health savings account (HSA).

I have included a list of available and vetted companies online at *www.BusyBrainCure.com* for you. If you do receive these laboratory evaluations, I will recommend that the long-term management of an abnormality in MTHFR deficiency, thyroid hormones, vitamin D3, or insulin resistance will need supervision from a medical professional.

This book and online program are not meant to replace medical care but rather to augment your healing and give you tools to take to your physician.

17

brainSHIFT Protocol, Week 8
Putting It All Together

Kevin first walked into our integrative medicine clinic in 2015; his anxiety and, to be honest, his negativity made it challenging for him to focus while I asked him basic questions so I could fill out his intake form. He was having conflict within all his relationships and shifting the blame for his life falling apart to his baby mama drama, his current wife, and the NBA client he had been managing. His life predicaments were everyone else's fault, clear back to his extended family in rural Georgia. Kevin was already working with a nutritionist and personal trainer and told me, "I'm eating clean, pumping iron, and dressing to the nines." I was sure that using the words *anxiety, insomnia, anger,* and *burnout* would be a further assault on his psyche, and frankly, I thought he would walk out of the clinic and write me off as another crazy and difficult person in his life.

But he persisted in his work with me over the next 2 months

as we recalibrated his sleep-wake cycle, assessed labs, and treated the underlying cause of his neuroinflammation. It's no surprise that once his mood and sleep were stabilized, the anger toward the people in his life subsided. He was able to come to an agreement on custody with his daughter's mother, and he not only stayed in his current marriage but worked with a relationship counselor to improve communication and romance. We continued to assess his attitudes toward his relationships and life with mindfulness-based cognitive therapy.

We also addressed labs such as his low vitamin D levels to maintain his health. In addition to taking vitamin D3, he managed his symptoms, continuing the supplement regimen we fine-tuned, being disciplined about sleep, and having a mindfulness practice.

I didn't have the term *Busy Brain* yet, nor had I started to research the vast medical literature as I have for this book and our online program. I was treating Kevin with the traditional integrative medicine protocols and additional mindfulness-based cognitive therapy. I began to see a pattern in the hundreds of cases like Kevin's in my clinical practice and through executive coaching.

From time to time, Kevin would show back up in the clinic when a new life challenge faced him (a Busy Brain can return with new stressors). On one of these occasions, it was his newborn baby that had him at his original levels of anxiety. My Aunties and medical training taught me well; I stood my ground and fussed, "Your wife just had a baby and hasn't slept a full night in 2 months. What are you doing to help support her? We have come too far in your care the last 2 years for you to go backward now."

He sat down. "Whoa, no one has taught me about this, Auntie, I mean, Dr. Auntie Romie."

He had shifted from a Busy Brain full of resistance to a sponge wanting to heal. He would now come to the clinic every few months for a checkup, and mostly to have a cup of chai with Auntie to catch up and give him blunt directions, *muh mitha karo*, of course, when needed.

When I was still seeing patients like Kevin in the integrative medicine clinic in Orlando, I didn't have the name *brainSHIFT Protocol* yet. Often, going through this entire treatment protocol with an individual could take months. We did not have the technology platforms and processes streamlined as we do now. Kevin named the process, "Dr. Auntie magic with a whole lotta tough straight talk."

When executive teams would hire me to work with them to help stress levels and optimize health, I would walk into their companies with large binders the size of medical books. The blessing of the global pandemic was that now companies, organizations, and individuals were reaching out with increased awareness about mental health and workplace wellness. We had this opportunity to build and scale the protocol online that had already helped countless other individuals and me heal our Busy Brains.

brainSHIFT

Congratulations on making it to the final week of the brainSHIFT Protocol. Now, if you were skimming section three to cherry-pick what felt easy, I'll lovingly and bluntly invite you to join me back at chapter 10 to start taking action, one brainSHIFT at a time.

Remember from chapter 10, it is time to face the triplets—resistance, denial, and projection—the three defense mechanisms dressed up as your Busy Brain's best friends who will prevent you from digging deeper, doing the work, and facing your fears.

Now I will ask you to look back at the health goal you wrote for yourself in chapter 10. How do you feel? Are you sleeping through the night? Did your belly bloating reduce? Are you feeling energized, even when you come home after a full, productive day of work?

We want to help you assess your progress. Remember the Busy Brain Test? We welcome you to take a few minutes to repeat it by going to *www.BusyBrainCure.com* and taking it for free.

When we look at the over 1,000 individuals who have gone through the brainSHIFT program prior to the submission of this book, we found the following improvement in individual scores:

- Sleep improved by 40%

- Physical symptoms improved by an average of 22%

- Emotional management improved by 20%

- Behavioral management improved by 17%

- Personal habits improved by 15%

What does this translate into? That individuals and teams slept better and had improved physical health in under 8 weeks.

Below is a list of all of the brainSHIFTs that stack upon each other week after week to cure your Busy Brain and help to alleviate burnout.

- How many were you able to try?

- Did any of them stick?

brainSHIFTs Weeks 1 through 8 Summary

Remember, brainSHIFTs build upon each other or stack each week. Here is a summary of the microhabits or brainSHIFTs we have started so far:

1. **Week 1 brainSHIFT:** Set a specific goal and outcome you desire for your 8-week brainSHIFT journey.

2. **Week 2 brainSHIFT:** Set a regular time to sleep at night and wake up each morning.

3. **Week 3 brainSHIFT:** It's time to add digital detox 30 to 60 minutes before bedtime. Find other calming rituals to replace screen time before sleep.

4. **Week 4 brainSHIFT:** Schedule a brainPAUSE for 3 minutes during the day and before bedtime.

5. **Week 5 brainSHIFT:** This week, you are avoiding high glycemic foods (white sugar, white flour, white potatoes, white rice, and white bread) within 1 hour of consuming caffeine.

6. **Week 6 brainSHIFT:** This week, you are making a list of healthy fats you enjoy eating and adding one to two servings of healthy fats to each meal.

7. **Week 7 brainSHIFT:** Talk to your primary care provider about checking your labs to assess your overall health and well-being with a special focus on your vitamin D levels.

8. **Week 8 brainSHIFT:** Repeat the Busy Brain Test. Look at your goals. Where is your score now?

brainWORK Week 8

1. This week, we will ask you to repeat the Busy Brain Test so you can see where you have improved. You can go to this link: *www.BusyBrainCure.com*.

2. I want you to take a look at all of the brainSHIFTs from weeks 1 through 8. The average number of brainSHIFTs individuals take forward is two or three—yet they still see remarkable healing! Give yourself grace if you were unable to try them all or stick with them.

3. If you haven't already, can you pick one brainSHIFT to continue past the 8 weeks? Share with us on social media, tagging me @drromie using hashtag #brainSHIFT. We want to hear your wins.

Wait, My Busy Brain Came Back Again. Did My Brain Fail Me?

Life happens, and as you saw with Kevin, new challenges can bring up our old patterns of a Busy Brain. This does not mean your health has deteriorated or that you are failing at life. You just might need a reminder from a loving Dr. Auntie in your life to brainSHIFT. Don't let your mind play tricks on you if you wake up at 2:37 a.m. with worries having hijacked a peaceful night of sleep. You lose focus in the middle of an important meeting at work or can't put your phone down because you are doomscrolling...or looking for more feel-good reels about organizing kitchen drawers.

Here are a few signs that you may need to revisit the brainSHIFT 8-week program:

- Waking up in the middle of the night worried.

- Wearing stress as a badge of honor.

- Feeling low-level anxious all day long.

- Being unable to shut down work before bedtime.

We typically find that people fit one of two teams when they slip back into a temporary Busy Brain:

1. I Can't Sleep Team

2. Who Stole My Energy Team

If you are team number one, start with brainSHIFTs weeks 1 to 4.

If you are sleeping fine but are playing on team two, go through weeks 4 through 8 again.

This book and the online community are available for you, and you can join others with a Busy Brain and cycle through whenever you feel the need. Auntie always has her living room ready to invite guests. We have removed the plastic from the sofa, the chai is warm, and comfort food is always welcomed.

As we come to the close of this book, you might be wondering: Hey, Dr. Auntie Romie, how do I know that I have cured my Busy Brain? Here are the telltale signs:

- You wake up feeling energized.

- You feel focused during your workday.

- You lead with calm consciousness.

- You have clear boundaries between home and work.

- You're able to be present with your loved ones.

I have to say, there are no coincidences when we live a life of service. As I finished writing this book to submit to my publisher, my iPhone dinged with a new message:

Rooooooommmmmieeee—can you feel the joy in my message? I have so many projects in the works to help NBA players and teams, and here is a picture of my baby girl that will make you smile.

My heart is filled with light and hope when I get these text message updates from Kevin. He is a recovering Busy Brained

DR. ROMIE MUSHTAQ

executive who, 5 years after last seeing me in the clinic, has used brainSHIFT to rebuild his business and, more importantly, his relationships. He is living a life of purpose, one driven by hope.

I know why I worked so hard to get this message out to you. Ask my team, and my senior dog Rahja. It's been a lot of early mornings to squeeze in writing while scaling a business that serves our mission. I wanted to share the Busy Brain Cure with you because I remember that dark feeling. I remember what it was like to feel alone at work at my first medical job, when no one asked how I was doing despite the fact that I was visibly ill and emotionally distraught. I thought I had failed as a doctor, daughter, and female leader. There was no fancy outfit, expensive dark chocolate, or luxe vacation package that could mask the fact that I was not only lonely, but also had lost complete hope.

I can't help but wonder what path my life would be on if I had only known then what I know now. And yet I would not have chosen that path, because I was meant to journey with you. Had I not burned out and needed surgery (and puked on my Prada), I would not have journeyed to meet global healers like the shaman in Guatemala or the compassionate giggling monk in Phnom Penh. I would not have had the courage to walk into Evolution Hospitality with a harebrained research idea, and walk out as Dr. Auntie Romie (Chief Wellness Officer) to all of our Evolutionaries.

Here is a confession you don't expect to read from me, your guide, the author of *The Busy Brain Cure*.

My Busy Brain still returns at the most inopportune times.

After years of research for this book and working with my developmental editor, Melanie, for a year to write the first draft, this book almost didn't make it to the finish line. I was delayed sending in the edits to the book to my editorial team at Hanover Square Press because my own Busy Brain returned. I was self-checking all the science, wondering if I had the right blend of story/science/action. I also wanted the "perfect" way to close this book for everyone who made it to the end (or turned to the back of the book to see how the story ends). I would then try to focus on the suggested edits throughout the rest of this book, and I would hear the old voices of judgmental Aunties in my mind—jeering at me.

Who are you to think you can share all of our stories so publicly? No one is going to read this book.

You wasted months on this book when you should have been running your business…you are a failure yet again.

You are always dreaming too big for a simple divorced Desi girl.

One thing was different this time compared to the young doctor crying in her sedan 16 years ago as I struggled to face another day of a job I loved that didn't always love me back. I recognized the symptoms and knew I didn't have to walk the journey alone. I hit the pause button and restarted the cycle of the 8-week brainSHIFT Protocol myself. I didn't do it alone, either; I had the accountability of my therapist, Karen, and my business coach, Pam, by my side. I took an 8-week break from writing this book to refocus on my role as Chief Wellness Officer at Evolution Hospitality—and be with the people with whom I started this initial research. I made a point to connect to friends and extended family members who I pushed away for many years while I prioritized to-do lists over people. I savored comfort food in the Bengali restaurants of Brick Lane in London. I danced with new friends at Lizzo's concert in Palm Springs as she wrapped up her "Special" tour—and stayed up in my stilettos way past my scheduled bedtime.

I had to live through what I am asking you to understand now: your Busy Brain never completely disappears. The to-do list items, people, and news cycles that once triggered a Busy Brain disappear and could be replaced by new stressors. We all must remember that you are human and not perfect. Perfection is in sitting with the imperfections of life. This book was written for all of us, the thousands of us who conquer one life goal or project at work and have seventeen more lined up.

As a human recovering from cycles of my own Busy Brain and burnout, the important thing I want you to know is that you are not alone. A Busy Brain will fool you into thinking that you are the only one that has lost control. A voice of judgment may also take over your spirit. Come back to the 8-week plan, and join the online community at *www.BusyBrainCure.com*.

As a physician, healer, and Chief Wellness Officer, I ask you to open your heart as a leader. The person who has suboptimal performance on your team, or is pissing you off, needs one thing from you: compassion.

The only way we replace judgment in our brains and toxicity in the workplace is to first brainSHIFT. When we tame our Busy Brains, we then lead our lives and teams with a calm, focused mind and, more importantly, an open heart.

I shared with you the stories and wisdom of my elders, Aunties, mentors, friends, and strangers who held hope for me during that trying time. As I journeyed to create this brain-SHIFT program, I learned from my Aunties how to be your hope-holder. I had the honor of holding hope for individuals like Kevin, Lorraine, Melanie, Nancy, and all the corporate teams who have joined us on this journey of a team brain-SHIFT program.

What do I have today, having learned to repeat this cycle of brainSHIFT? Hope. And as for how the story ends—well, that nonsense is for the fairy tales. Our story together is just starting.

When I choose to brainSHIFT, my mind stays focused and calm.

My heart stays open, a place of compassion for all whom I serve, and most of all, for myself.

And, well, I still hope that by the time this book makes it to print, I have a second chance at love from a companion in my life.

I hope to continue to find a way to uplift the next generation of women and girls—the future STEMinists.

Tell me, what is one hope you have for yourself?

When I ask this question at the end of my lectures, people often tell me their hopes for their children, partners, or companies, but what I really want to know about is your personal hope for your brain, body, and life.

When we face our Busy Brain and choose to brainSHIFT, we are able to succeed at a level we never realized while living a life of purpose.

That is my fervent hope for all of you.

Who could you be?
What can you achieve?
It all starts with a brainSHIFT.
We are in this together. Let's brainSHIFT.

—*Dr. Romie*

APPENDIX A

Chapter 2 and Chapter 10: Take the Busy Brain Test

How to take the Busy Brain Test and obtain your score:

Go to *www.BusyBrainCure.com* to take the Busy Brain Test for free.

Alternatively, you can scan this QR code with the camera on your phone or tablet and be directed to the same link:

Chapter 16: brainSHIFT Protocol Laboratory Evaluations

Go to *www.BusyBrainCure.com* and in our free resources, you can download the laboratory evaluation forms to take to your physician.

In addition, I am listing the key laboratory evaluations here that are done with your doctor's orders at a lab where blood can be drawn.

Evaluation of your vitamin D levels:

1. Complete blood count

2. Serum 25-hydroxyvitamin D test

Evaluation of your thyroid gland function:

1. TSH

2. Total T4

3. Total T3

4. Free T4

5. Free T3

6. Reverse T3

7. Thyroid Peroxidase Antibodies

8. Anti-Thyroglobulin Antibodies

Evaluation of markers of inflammation:

1. Hemoglobin A1c (HbA1c)

2. Morning serum cortisol level

3. Serum homocysteine levels

4. High sensitivity C-reactive protein (hS-CRP)

APPENDIX B

What can I eat during the brainSHIFT 8-Week Protocol?

Go to *www.BusyBrainCure.com* and in our free resources, you will find our food suggestions for weeks 5 through 8 of the brainSHIFT Protocol.

brainSHIFT Week 5

During week 5 of the brainSHIFT Protocol, we ask you to try to incorporate more low glycemic index foods into your meals. Now remember, comfort food is still allowed. We just ask that you schedule your comfort food meals 1–2 times a week during the 8-week protocol.

Low-Glycemic Fruit

• Apples

- Dried apricots

- Underripe bananas

- Peaches

- Strawberries

- Oranges

- Cherries

- Coconut

- Cranberries

- Blueberries

- Pears

- Plums

- Grapefruit

Low-Glycemic Vegetables

- Carrots

- Green peas

- Onions

- Lettuce

- Greens (spinach, kale, collards, beet)

- Green beans

- Tomatoes

- Cucumbers

- Bok choy

- Mushrooms

- Artichokes

- Brussels sprouts

- Cabbage

- Broccoli

- Cauliflower

- Celery

- Eggplant

- Peppers (bell peppers, jalapeños, serrano, etc.)

- Zucchini and crookneck squash

- Snow peas

Low-Glycemic Grains

- Barley

- Whole wheat kernels

- All-Bran and Fiber One cereals

- Oat bran and rice bran cereals

- Whole grain pasta

- Lasagna with meat and/or cheese, ravioli, tortellini, and other stuffed pasta

- Whole grain pumpernickel bread

- Sourdough bread

- Wheat tortilla

Low-Glycemic Dairy Products and Dairy-Substitute Products

- Skim, low-fat, and whole milk

- Plain yogurt

- Cheese (cheddar, Swiss, mozzarella, Brie, feta, blue, goat, etc.)

- Cottage cheese

- Ricotta cheese

- Soy milk and yogurt

Low-Glycemic Legumes

- Beans (chickpeas, kidney beans, pinto beans, black beans, navy beans, etc.)

- Lima beans

- Split peas, black-eyed peas

- Lentils

- Edamame and roasted soybeans

- Hummus

- Bean dip

- Tofu and soy-based meat substitutes

brainSHIFT Week 6

During week 6 of the brainSHIFT Protocol, we ask you to try to incorporate 1–2 servings of healthy fats at each meal. Now remember, comfort food is still allowed. We just ask that you schedule your comfort food meals 1–2 times a week during the 8-week protocol.

Healthy Fats

- Avocados

- Cheese

- Dark chocolate (at least 70% dark chocolate, be mindful of added sugar)

- Whole eggs (yes, include the yolk)

- Fatty fish (salmon, mackerel, tuna)

- Nuts (almonds, walnuts, pecans)

- Chia seeds

- Oils (extra virgin olive oil, avocado oil, grapeseed oil, ghee, coconut oil)

- Full-fat yogurt

APPENDIX C

Comfort Food Recipes

In the Busy Brain Cure, the goal is to heal your Busy Brain so we can minimize stress. As a doctor, Chief Wellness Officer, and woman of a diverse background, I strongly stand in opposition of the American fad diet culture for two reasons:

1. While I believe in eating "anti-inflammatory" foods, too often these diets only promote foods that fail to honor diversity and inclusion. These diets do not account for foods associated with religious holidays, family traditions, ethnic background, home states, or country of origin.

2. Diets fail because the foods our brains associate with joy and memories of loved ones are labeled as "bad for us to eat." Our brains then have raised stress levels, guilt, and shame to replace the joy of a meal.

In honor of my elders, I am sharing a few of our favorite comfort food recipes, and you can find even more at *www. BusyBrainCure.com.*

Traditional Chai for Aunties' Afternoon Tea Party

Note: There was a lot of debate from my Aunties about the spices and type of milk to use. To be a peacekeeper, I am sharing my variation.

Ingredients

1. Tapal Danedar or Ahmad Tea—1 ½ tsp loose leaf tea for every cup

2. 1 ¼ cup water

3. 1 cup whole milk

4. 1–2 green cardamon pods (not the black cardamon)

Substitute coconut milk or almond milk if you avoid dairy.

I add fresh ginger to aid with digestion when my stomach is upset.

I add a cinnamon stick when I need a little boost of joy.

Instructions

1. In a medium saucepan, bring the water to a boil, then add in tea leaves and cardamon.

2. Reduce the heat to medium and allow to simmer for 1–2 minutes.

3. Add the milk and raise the heat to high and allow to boil.

4. As it begins to boil, the chai will rise in the saucepan. Remove the pan from the heat before the tea reaches the top of the saucepan. Do this a few times to allow ingredients to blend while using a ladle to scoop and pour back the chai. Alternately, once it comes to a boil, lower the heat and allow it to simmer to the desired strength (typically 3–5 minutes).

5. Pour the chai through a small sieve into your favorite cup and sweeten using stevia if necessary.

Nanni's Punjabi Chicken Biryani Recipe

My maternal grandmother (Nanni) was a gifted chef and the queen of her kitchen; you could taste her love and healing intentions in every meal she cooked. When she made her biryani recipe, the aroma would fill the entire street, and neighbors would gather to share in the delight. She didn't use proper measurements, just her intuition when adding a pinch or bunch of ingredients. This recipe is as close as I could create while feeling her presence looking down from Heaven.

Prep and cook time: The recipe books say 3 hours—it took me 2 days, and a third to clean up the mess.

Ingredients

For the meat mixture:

- 1 lb. chicken (you can also use mutton)
- Ghee (clarified butter)
- 1 large onion, sliced
- 3 large tomatoes, diced
- 1 tbsp ground/grated fresh ginger
- 1 tbsp ground/crushed fresh garlic
- ½ cup whole milk yogurt
- 2 tsp salt
- 1 tbsp red chili powder
- ½ tsp turmeric power
- ½ tsp crushed coriander seeds
- ½ tsp cumin
- ½ tsp fennel seeds (saunf)
- 2 large black cardamom seeds
- 4 green cardamom seeds
- 2 small cinnamon sticks

- 6–7 whole black peppercorns

- Generous handfuls of chopped fresh coriander leaves or cilantro leaves

- 3–4 green chilies

Pro tip: My modern-day Punjabi sisters will tell you to skip a few hours in the kitchen and use Shan Masala premixed spice packages.

For the rice:

- 3 cups basmati rice, rinsed and soaked

- 1 tbsp vinegar

- 2 generous tsp salt

Instructions

Meat preparation:

1. Slice your onions and cook in ghee in a large pot till browned.

2. Put in the ginger, garlic, and tomatoes and cook until it is a chunky sauce.

3. Add the yogurt, remaining spices, meat, and green chilies. Stir and mix well.

4. If using chicken, add one cup of hot water, bring to a boil,

then simmer till tender. For tougher meats, i.e. mutton, add more water.

5. Add coriander (or cilantro) leaves.

Rice preparation:

1. In a large pot, add water, salt, and vinegar to the soaked rice and boil until it is parboiled, i.e. most of the grain is translucent with an opaque center.

2. Strain the rice when done.

Final step in cooking the biryani:

1. In a large pot, grease the bottom with ghee.

2. Layer the rice in the following order: half the rice, all the meat masala, remaining rice, and leave on the lowest heat setting for 15–20 minutes.

Note: In India and Pakistan, the rice is often yellow because of food coloring. I omitted that step as I couldn't find a natural yellow food coloring that didn't alter the taste of the rice.

Sarson ka Saag Recipe in Loving Memory of Mrs. Shaista Anjum

My favorite memory of Shaista Aunty is that she always brought laughter and happiness to the room, especially when I was overwhelmed with life's problems. In memory of Shaista Aunty, her daughter, Shamela, shares her adapted version of

Sarson ka Saag, a Punjabi dish made of mustard greens, spinach, fenugreek leaves, and spices.

Ingredients

- 1 lb. mustard greens (sarson)

- ½ lb. spinach

- ½ bunch fenugreek leaves (methi)

- 1 jalapeño pepper, diced

- 1 serrano pepper, diced

- 1 tbsp garlic paste

- ½ tbsp ginger paste

- 1 tsp cumin seeds

- 1 tsp coriander powder

- ½ large red onion, diced

- 1 large vine tomato, diced

- ¼ cup oil

- ½ cup water

Add after greens have cooked/softened:

- 1 tsp garam masala

- 1 ½ tsp salt

- 1 tbsp butter

- ½ tsp dried fenugreek leaves (kasouri methi)

For tempering the saag (tadka):

- ¼ cup oil

- 4 cloves of garlic, crushed

Instructions

1. Thoroughly wash all the greens several times under running water and then chop them up into fine small pieces.

2. In a large pot on low medium heat, add all the ingredients in the first list and cover.

3. Cook for about 30 minutes until the greens have cooked through and softened.

4. Let the mixture cool and then transfer it to a blender and pulse to the desired consistency, being careful not to over-blend.

5. Transfer it all back to the cooking pot used previously and turn the heat to low.

6. Now add the second ingredient list of garam masala, salt, butter, and dried fenugreek leaves.

7. Cook for 5–10 minutes, stirring regularly to prevent the saag from sticking to the bottom.

8. If the saag is too thick, additional boiled water can be added at this time but add only a little at a time.

9. For tempering, in a separate frying pan, add oil and crushed garlic and cook on medium heat.

10. Once garlic comes to a medium brown color, add to the saag mixture and simmer for 5 minutes.

11. Garnish with more butter and enjoy!

Ami's Savaiya in Loving Memory of Dr. Shameema Zaheer

Aunty Shameema was my aunty who shared a love of fabulous high heels, desserts, and breaking the glass ceiling as a woman in medicine in the 1950s. She always had a prayer for me to use to center my Busy Brain. Her daughter, Ayesha, is one of my childhood best friends and shared Ami's savaiya.

From Ayesha:

Ami means mother in Urdu. So this is my mother's recipe. Savaiya is a sweet dish that is traditionally served as a dessert. It is also a special "breakfast porridge" that is served on Eid ul Fitr, a celebration after fasting for 30 days from sunrise to sunset during the month of Ramadan. This dish marks the end of the fasting month and was always on our table for Eid breakfast before we left for holiday prayers, and it was eaten throughout the day celebrating with family and friends.

Ingredients

- 3 oz. of vermicelli

- 1 stick of butter (or ghee)

- 6 cups of half and half

- ¼ tsp of cardamon seeds

- ¼ cup of chopped almonds or pistachios

- 2 tbsp of golden raisins

- 6–8 oz. of sugar (depending on how sweet you like desserts)

Instructions

1. Warm the half and half in a heavy-bottom saucepan with cardamon seeds on low heat.

2. Melt butter in a separate 6- or 8-quart stockpot over medium-low heat.

3. Break vermicelli into 2- or 3-inch-long pieces and add to the stockpot with the melted butter.

4. Sauté the vermicelli frequently on medium-low heat until it turns golden brown.

5. Add the warmed-up half and half to the vermicelli and bring to a slow simmer.

6. Add golden raisins and chopped almonds or pistachios.

7. Continue to cook the vermicelli and half and half on medium, stirring frequently until the mixture thickens and starts to stick to your stirring spoon (about 20–30 minutes).

8. When thickened like a porridge (or to the consistency you like), add sugar and cook for another 5 minutes.

9. Pour into a serving bowl and garnish with more chopped almonds or pistachios.

Mamaw's Southern Chicken & Dumplings

Melissa Deloach Mart is one of my sister-friends who was my lifeline during the long years of residency training in South Carolina. She and her mother, Diann, have been in my life with Southern Aunty wisdom ever since.

From Melissa:

Growing up in the South, nothing was more comforting than a Sunday supper with a big hearty bowl of my grandmother's famous chicken & dumplings. I remember her making it seem so effortless, every cloudlike dumpling crafted with love. Feeding others is how my grandmother soothed her own Busy Brain. Of course, Mamaw didn't have a recipe. Everything she made was done by "feel"—a little bit of this and a whole lot of that (typically butter). Over the years, my aunts, cousins, and I have made this version of chicken and dumplings from our memory of the ingredients and the process we observed. I can't say if it's precisely how Mamaw made it, but the sight, sound, and satisfying taste of this recipe sure feel like the comfort of her Southern kitchen.

Ingredients

For the chicken:

- 1 whole chicken, about 3.5–5 lbs.

- 1 ½ tsp salt

- 8 cups water

For the dumplings:

- 2 cups self-rising flour

- 1 heaping tbsp shortening (Crisco brand was Mamaw's favorite)

- ½ cup buttermilk

- ½ cup cold water

For the sauce:

- 1 stick of butter

- 12 oz. can evaporated milk

- ½ tbsp black pepper

- Salt to taste

Instructions

1. Place the chicken in a large Dutch oven and cover with water. Bring the chicken to a boil over medium heat, then reduce to low and cook until tender, approximately 2 hours.

2. Remove the chicken and shred into tiny strips. Remove 2 cups of broth. Set both aside. Add salt to the broth, increase the heat, and bring to a boil.

3. To make the dumplings, mix flour, shortening, buttermilk, and cold water together to form a dough. Do not overwork the dough.

4. Pour the dough onto a lightly floured surface and roll out to ½-inch thickness. Pinch off dough pieces and gently form 2-inch balls. Drop the dough pieces into the boiling broth. Gently stir the dumplings occasionally to make sure they are submerged in the broth.

5. Add the chicken back into the broth. Add the butter and evaporated milk, stirring to combine. Allow to gently boil for 3–5 more minutes. To test for doneness, remove a dumpling, cut it in half, and check the dough. It should be firm but slightly moist in the middle.

6. Season the sauce with black pepper and additional salt to taste. If the sauce is too thick, gradually add in the reserved chicken broth and stir.

7. Allow the chicken and dumplings to rest 10–15 minutes before serving.

Mandy's Roast Beef Gravy and Biscuits Recipe

Mandy Allen is the brainSHIFT Institute's online business manager and design director.

From Mandy:

My grandmother started making roast beef gravy for breakfast during the Great Depression to stretch meals to feed their large family of eight. Grandmother mentioned many times how if it wasn't for her resourcefulness, crops, and farm animals that they did have, they would have truly gone hungry.

The recipe is based on one can of roast beef and gravy found at the grocery store near canned chicken, tuna, etc. Our family's preferred brands are Hereford or Libby. Grandmother would stretch this by making a larger roux, adding more water, and still only using one can of roast beef. She always said to toast the flour in the roux to a golden brown to add flavor. Typically served over biscuits but we've been known to eat it on top of freshly toasted bread.

Ingredients

- 12 oz. can roast beef with gravy

- 3 tbsp Crisco, butter, or oil of choice

- 3 tbsp self-rising flour

- 2 cups water

- Salt and pepper to taste

Instructions

1. Begin the gravy with a roux consisting of the Crisco and flour. Open the can of roast beef and gravy and, using the can lid as a strainer, strain out the gravy and add to the Crisco mixture to aid in creating the roux portion of the gravy.

2. Cook the roux until the flour is browned. The darker the color of flour, the nuttier the flavor.

3. Add water until you reach the desired gravy consistency. We like our gravy a bit on the thicker side (think sausage gravy) but it is good as long as it coats the back of a spoon.

4. Take the roast beef meat from the can and, using clean hands, separate and flake the meat and add into the gravy.

5. Add salt and pepper to taste.

6. Allow to simmer for 5 minutes, stirring frequently to prevent sticking.

7. Serve warm over split-open buttermilk biscuits.

Pesto Pritchardi: From the Kitchen of the Late Dr. Paul B. Pritchard III

No matter where I am in the world, whenever someone utters the word "pesto," I think of Dr. Paul B. Pritchard III and his wife, Rebecca. In his memory, his daughter, Nancy Pritchard Jackson, shared his recipe.

Ingredients

- 1 cup virgin olive oil
- 1 cup fresh basil leaves
- 1 cup lightly toasted pine nuts
- ¼ tsp salt
- ⅛ tsp ground pepper
- 1 cup freshly ground parmesan cheese

Instructions

1. Toast the pine nuts on medium heat in a skillet without oil. Caution: Don't burn the pine nuts!

2. Gently tear the basil into small pieces and place into a blender with oil. Mix well on medium speed.

3. Turn off the blender and mix parmesan into the blender using a mixing spoon.

4. Then add salt, pepper, and the toasted pine nuts. Mix well in the blender.

Swedish Meatballs from the Kitchen of Melanie Bates

Melanie Bates is not only my developmental editor but also a self-proclaimed "Farm Aunty."

From Melanie:

On special occasions like my birthday, my mom would let me choose what we would have for dinner, and, for me, there was never any question. It was always Swedish meatballs.

These days, Swedish meatballs are still my go-to comfort food. I follow Alton Brown's recipe, which you can find online on Food Network, and everything is homemade. For clarified butter, I use ghee, and instead of Minute Rice, I cook basmati in my rice cooker. I've also been known to sub beef bone broth in place of regular beef broth.

Ingredients

- 2 slices fresh white bread

- ¼ cup milk

- 3 tbsp ghee (clarified butter), divided

- ½ cup finely chopped onion

- A pinch plus 1 tsp kosher salt

- ¾ lb. ground chuck

- ¾ lb. ground pork

- 2 large egg yolks

- ½ tsp black pepper

- ¼ tsp ground allspice

- ¼ tsp freshly grated nutmeg

- ¼ cup all-purpose flour

- 3 cups beef broth

- ¼ cup heavy cream

Instructions

1. Preheat oven to 200 degrees F.

2. Tear the bread into pieces and place in a small mixing bowl along with the milk. Set aside.

3. In a 12-inch straight-sided sauté pan over medium heat, melt 1 tablespoon of the butter. Add the onion and a pinch of salt and sweat until the onions are soft. Remove from the heat and set aside.

4. In the bowl of a stand mixer, combine the bread and milk mixture, ground chuck, pork, egg yolks, 1 teaspoon of kosher salt, black pepper, allspice, nutmeg, and onions. Beat on medium speed for 1–2 minutes.

5. Using a scale, weigh meatballs into 1-ounce portions and

place on a sheet pan. Using your hands, shape the meat-balls into rounds.

6. Heat the remaining butter in the sauté pan over medium-low heat, or in an electric skillet set to 250 degrees F. Add the meatballs and sauté until golden brown on all sides, about 7–10 minutes.

7. Move the meatballs to an ovenproof dish using a slotted spoon and place in the warmed oven.

8. Once all of the meatballs are cooked, decrease the heat to low and add the flour to the pan or skillet. Whisk until lightly browned, approximately 1–2 minutes. Gradually add the beef stock and whisk until the sauce begins to thicken. Add the cream and cook until the gravy reaches the desired consistency.

9. Remove the meatballs from the oven, cover with the gravy, and serve.

Cochran Skyline Chili from the Kitchen of Karen Smith Cochran

Karen is a sister-friend whose kitchen provided me with many comfort food meals while I researched and wrote this book. The chili is one of our favorites from her family recipe book.

From Karen:

This recipe is a comfort food staple in our home. We use ground turkey instead of hamburger. The chili is eaten over spaghetti and topped with your favorite fixins'—sour cream, shredded cheddar cheese, onions—with a bottle of hot sauce on the side for those who desire a bit of heat.

Ingredients

- 1 ½ lbs. hamburger or ground turkey

- 1 medium onion, chopped

- 1 tsp chili powder

- 5–6 cans of tomato sauce (8 oz.)

- 2 cans of kidney beans (16 oz.)

- 2 dashes of Tabasco

- Salt to taste

Additional ingredients:

- 1 box of spaghetti

- Sour cream

- Shredded cheddar cheese

- Diced onions for garnish

Instructions

1. Cook onion and ground meat until meat is cooked through; drain.

2. Add tomato sauce, chili powder, Tabasco, and salt. Cook for ½ hour.

3. Add kidney beans—do NOT drain. Continue to cook until beans are warmed through, approximately 10 minutes.

4. In a separate pot, prepare spaghetti according to package directions.

When ready to serve, fill a bowl with spaghetti and top with chili.

Add fixins' and enjoy!

Charlie's Brexit Potato Casserole from the
Kitchen of Charles Smith

Charlie Smith is a friend from Florida who retired and moved to the countryside of France. He suddenly found himself divorced, a bachelor, and sought to comfort himself by growing flowers and cooking with fresh ingredients from the market in his kitchen.

Note: This is a different Charles from the one in chapter 11.

Ingredients

- 2 ½ cups of thickly sliced French waxy, yellow potatoes

- One medium yellow onion, diced

- 4 peeled garlic cloves (the number coincides with your love of garlic)

- ¾ cup heavy, stabilized French cream

- 150 grams grated Wensleydale Cheddar Cheese—if you aren't near Neal's Yard Dairy in the UK, use an aged white cheddar-style cheese. Use more than you believe you should.

- Salt to taste

- Fresh ground black pepper to taste

Instructions

1. Preheat oven to 350 degrees F.

2. Assemble the potatoes, garlic, and onions in a roasting pan and toss loosely.

3. Pour the cream over the mixture, putting at least a drizzle on the top layer of vegetables.

4. Add seasoning to taste.

5. Cover evenly with the Wensleydale Cheese and place in the center rack of a warmed oven.

6. Cook at least 75 minutes or until the cheese top has started to turn a golden brown color—not all over; just in spots.

7. Remove from the oven and allow to cool slightly. Serve

with any meal you desire as a potato course—or eat it out of the pan!

This dish tastes better when allowed to cool, covered, and reheated later.

BIBLIOGRAPHY

Chapter 1

Liu, Xinyu, Yuhao Shan, Min Peng, Huanyu Chen, and Tong Chen. "Human Stress and StO2: Database, Features, and Classification of Emotional and Physical Stress." Entropy 22, no. 9 (2020): 962.

World Health Organization. "Occupational Stress, Burnout and Fatigue." Accessed April 24, 2023. *https://www.who.int/ tools/occupational-hazards-in-health-sector/occup-stress-burnout-fatigue.*

Brown, Theodore M., and Elizabeth Fee. "Walter Bradford Cannon: Pioneer Physiologist of Human Emotions." American Journal of Public Health 92, no. 10 (2002): 1594–95.

Koutsimani, Panagiota, Anthony Montgomery, and Katerina Georganta. "The Relationship Between Burnout, Depression, and Anxiety: A Systematic Review and Meta-Analysis." Frontiers in Psychology 10 (2019): 284.

Hong, Kan. "Classification of Emotional Stress and Physical Stress Using a Multispectral Based Deep Feature Extraction Model." Scientific Reports 13, no. 1 (2023): 2693.

López-Ibor, Juan J. "The Classification of Stress-Related Disorders in ICD-10 and DSM-IV." Psychopathology 35, no. 2–3 (2002): 107–11.

Smiljanic, Stasha. "21+ Statistics About The Health And Wellness Industry (2023)." PolicyAdvice, March 23, 2023. *https://policyadvice.net/insurance/insights/health-wellness-industry/*.

Gay, Charles. "Delta's History: From Dusting Crops to Connecting the World." Delta News Hub, April 23, 2019. *https://news.delta.com/deltas-history-dusting-crops-connecting-world*.

Chapter 2

Atroszko, Paweł A., Zsolt Demetrovics, and Mark D. Griffiths. "Work Addiction, Obsessive-Compulsive Personality Disorder, Burn-Out, and Global Burden of Disease: Implications from the ICD-11." International Journal of Environmental Research and Public Health 17, no. 2 (2020): 660.

"Tips for Coping with Stress." Centers for Disease Control and Prevention." Last reviewed November 30, 2021. *https://www.cdc.gov/violenceprevention/about/copingwith-stresstips.html*.

Dhama, K., S. K. Latheef, M. Dadar, H. A. Samad, A. Munjal, R. Khandia, and S. K. Joshi, et al. "Biomarkers in Stress Related Diseases/Disorders: Diagnostic, Prognostic, and Therapeutic Values." Frontiers in Molecular Biosciences 6 (2019): 91. DOI: 10.3389/fmolb.2019.00091.

Bazan, Nicolas G. "Neuroinflammation." Basic Neurochemistry: Principles of Molecular, Cellular, and Medical Neurobiology, edited by Scott Brady et al., 8th ed., 610–20. Waltham: Academic Press, 2012.

DiSabato, Damon J., Ning Quan, and Jonathan P. Godbout. "Neuroinflammation: The Devil Is in the Details." Journal of Neurochemistry 139, Suppl 2 (2016): 136–53.

Silver, Natalie. "Everything to Know About Your Circadian Rhythm." Healthline, March 30, 2022. https://www.healthline.com/health/healthy-sleep/circadian-rhythm.

Nicolaides, Nicolas C., Evangelia Charmandari, Tomoshige Kino, and George P. Chrousos. "Stress-Related and Circadian Secretion and Target Tissue Actions of Glucocorticoids: Impact on Health." Frontiers in Endocrinology 8 (2017): 70.

Oster, Henrik. "The Interplay between Stress, Biological Clocks and Metabolic Function." In Endocrine Abstracts, vol. 65. Society for Endocrinology BES 2019, Bioscientifica, 2019. S5.1.

Koch, Christiane E., B. Leinweber, B. C. Drengberg, C. Blaum, and H. Oster. "Interaction between Circadian Rhythms and Stress." Neurobiology of Stress 6 (2017): 57–67.

Keel, Peter. "Psychische Belastungen durch die Arbeit: Burnout-Syndrom [Psychological Stress Caused by Work: Burnout Syndrome]." Sozial-und Präventivmedizin 38, Suppl 2 (1993): S131–32.

"Workplace Stress." The American Institute of Stress, accessed April 24, 2023. https://www.stress.org/workplace-stress.

"State of the Global Workplace 2022 Report: The Voice of the World's Employees." Gallup, 2022. https://www.gallup.com/workplace/349484/state-of-the-global-workplace.aspx.

"Aflac WorkForces Report: 2022–2023." Aflac, 2023. https://www.aflac.com/business/resources/aflac-workforces-report/default.aspx.

Miklósi, M., O. Máté, K. Somogyi, and M. Szabó. "Adult attention deficit hyperactivity disorder symptoms, perceived stress, and well-being." The Journal of Nervous and Mental Disease 204 (2016): 364–9.

Calcia, M. A., D. R. Bonsall, P. S. Bloomfield, S. Selvaraj, T. Barichello, and O. D. Howes. "Stress and neuroinflammation: a systematic review of the effects of stress on microglia and the implications for mental illness." Psychopharmacology (Berl) 233(9) (2016): 1637–50. DOI: 10.1007/s00213-016-4218-9.

Ravi, Meghna, Andrew H. Miller, and Vasiliki Michopoulos. "The Immunology of Stress and the Impact of Inflammation on the Brain and Behaviour." BJPsych Advances 27, Suppl 3 (2021): 158–65.

Won, Eunsoo, and Yong-Ku Kim. "Neuroinflammation-Associated Alterations of the Brain as Potential Neural Biomarkers in Anxiety Disorders." International Journal of Molecular Sciences 21, no. 18 (2020): 6546.

Wang, Xiao-Lan, and Lianjian Li. "Circadian Clock Regulates Inflammation and the Development of Neurodegeneration." Frontiers in Cellular and Infection Microbiology 11 (2021): 696554.

Chapter 3

Research and Markets. "Workplace Stress Management Market: Global Industry Trends, Share, Size, Growth, Opportunity and Forecast 2023–2028." March 2023. https://www.researchandmarkets.com/reports/5769239/workplace-stress-management-market-global.

American Psychological Association (APA). "Stress in America 2022." Accessed April 2023. https://www.apa.org/news/press/releases/stress/2022/october-2022-questions.pdf.

"More Than a Quarter of U.S. Adults Say They're So Stressed They Can't Function." American Psychological Association, October 19, 2022. https://www.apa.org/news/press/releases/2022/10/multiple-stressors-no-function.

Abramson, Ashley. "Burnout and Stress Are Everywhere." Monitor on Psychology 53, no. 1 (2022): 72. https://www.apa.org/monitor/2022/01/special-burnout-stress.

"Depression Treatment After Unsatisfactory Response to

SSRIs When Used as First-Line Therapy." Effective Health Care Program-Agency for Healthcare Research and Quality, last reviewed December 2019, *https://effectivehealthcare.ahrq.gov/products/depression-treatment-ssri/research-protocol*.

Cassano, Giovanni B., Nicolò Baldini Rossi, and Stefano Pini. "Psychopharmacology of Anxiety Disorders." Dialogues in Clinical Neuroscience 4, no. 3 (2002): 271–85.

Sugarman, Michael A., Amy M. Loree, Boris B. Baltes, Emily R. Grekin, and Irving Kirsch. "The Efficacy of Paroxetine and Placebo in Treating Anxiety and Depression: A Meta-Analysis of Change on the Hamilton Rating Scales." PLoS One 9, no. 8 (2014): e106337.

Sartori, Simone B., and Nicolas Singewald. "Novel Pharmacological Targets in Drug Development for the Treatment of Anxiety and Anxiety-Related Disorders." Pharmacology & Therapeutics 204 (2019): 107402.

Rosnick, Christopher B., Julie L. Wetherell, Kamila S. White, Carmen Andreescu, David Dixon, and Eric J. Lenze. "Cognitive-Behavioral Therapy Augmentation of SSRI Reduces Cortisol Levels in Older Adults with Generalized Anxiety Disorder: A Randomized Clinical Trial." Journal of Consulting and Clinical Psychology 84, no. 4 (2016): 345–52.

Slee, April, Irwin Nazareth, Paulina Bondaronek, Yifeng Liu, Zhihang Cheng, and Nick Freemantle. "Pharmacological Treatments for Generalised Anxiety Disorder: A Systematic Review and Network Meta-Analysis." Lancet 393, no. 10173 (2019): 768–77.

Offidani, Emanuela, Jenny Guidi, Elena Tomba, and Giovanni Andrea Fava. "Efficacy and Tolerability of Benzodiazepines versus Antidepressants in Anxiety Disorders: A Systematic Review and Meta-Analysis." Psychotherapy and Psychosomatics 82, no. 6 (2013): 355–62.

Buscemi, Nina, Ben Vandermeer, Carol Friesen, Liza Bialy, Michelle Tubman, Maria Ospina, Terry P. Klassen, and Manisha Witmans. "The Efficacy and Safety of Drug Treatments for Chronic Insomnia in Adults: A Meta-Analysis of RCTs." Journal of General Internal Medicine 22, no. 9 (2007): 1335–50.

Chapter 4

LaFaver, K., J. M. Miyasaki, C. M. Keran, C. Rheaume, L. Gulya, K. H. Levin, E. C. Jones, H. B. Schwarz, J. R. Molano, A. Hessler, D. Singhal, T. D. Shanafelt, J. A. Sloan, P. J. Novotny, T. L. Cascino, and N. A. Busis. "Age and sex differences in burnout, career satisfaction, and well-being in US neurologists." Neurology 91, no. 20 (2018): e1928–e1941. https://doi.org/10.1212/WNL.0000000000006497.

Schlottmann, F., and M. G. Patti. "Esophageal achalasia: current diagnosis and treatment." Expert Review of Gastroenterology & Hepatology 12, no. 7 (2018): 711–21. https://doi.org/10.1080/17474124.2018.148174.

Millstine, D., C. Y. Chen, and B. Bauer. "Complementary and integrative medicine in the management of headache."

BMJ (Clinical Research Ed.) 357 (2017): j1805. *https://doi. org/10.1136/bmj.j1805.*

Maizes, V., D. Rakel, and C. Niemiec. "Integrative medicine and patient-centered care." Explore (New York, N.Y.) 5, no. 5 (2009): 277–289. *https://doi.org/10.1016/j.explore.2009.06.008.*

Fortney, L., D. Rakel, J. A. Rindfleisch, and J. Mallory. "Introduction to integrative primary care: the health-oriented clinic." Primary Care 37, no. 1 (2010): 1–12. *https://doi. org/10.1016/j.pop.2009.09.003.*

Adam, E. K., M. E. Quinn, R. Tavernier, M. T. McQuillan, K. A. Dahlke, and K. E. Gilbert. "Diurnal cortisol slopes and mental and physical health outcomes: A systematic review and meta-analysis." Psychoneuroendocrinology 83 (2017): 25–41. *https://doi.org/10.1016/j.psyneuen.2017.05.018.*

Jovanovski, Natalie, and Tess Jaeger. "Demystifying 'diet culture': Exploring the meaning of diet culture in online 'anti-diet' feminist, fat activist, and health professional communities." Women's Studies International Forum Volume 90 (2022): 102558. ISSN 0277-5395. *https://doi.org/10.1016/j. wsif.2021.102558.*

França, K., and T. M. Lotti. "Psycho-Neuro-Endocrine-Immunology: A Psychobiological Concept." Advances in Experimental Medicine and Biology 996 (2017): 123–34. *https:// doi.org/10.1007/978-3-319-56017-5_11.*

Bitzer-Quintero, O. K., et al. "Psycho-Neuro-Endocrine-Immunology: A Role for Melatonin in This New Paradigm."

Molecules (Basel, Switzerland) 27, no. 15 (2022): 4888. *https:// doi.org/10.3390/molecules27154888.*

Gonzalez-Diaz, S. N., A. Arias-Cruz, B. Elizondo-Villarreal, and O. P. Monge-Ortega. "Psychoneuroimmunoendocrinology: Clinical implications." World Allergy Organization Journal 10 (2017): 19. DOI: 10.1186/s40413-017-0151-6.

Bottaccioli, F., and A. G. Bottaccioli. "Nervous regulation." In Psycho-Neuro-Endocrine-Immunology and Science of the Integrated Care the Manual, edited by F. Bottaccioli, A. G. Bottaccioli. Edra S.p.A., Milano, Italy, 2020, pp. 103–26.

Daniel, P. M. "Anatomy of the hypothalamus and pituitary gland." Journal of Clinical Pathology: Supplement (Association of Clinical Pathologists) 7 (1976): 1–7. DOI: 10.1136/ jcp.s1-7.1.1.

Bottaccioli, F., and A. G. Bottaccioli. "Neuroendocrine regulation." Psycho-Neuro-Endocrine-Immunology and Science of the Integrated Care the Manual, edited by F. Bottaccioli, A. G. Bottaccioli. Edra S.p.A., Milano, Italy, 2020, pp. 131–51.

Feldt-Rasmussen, U., G. Effraimidis, and M. Klose. "The hypothalamus-pituitary-thyroid (HPT)-axis and its role in physiology and pathophysiology of other hypothalamus-pituitary functions." Molecular and Cellular Endocrinology 525 (2021): 111173. DOI: 10.1016/j.mce.2021.111173.

Alizadeh, M., A. Mirzazadeh, D. X. Parmelee, E. Peyton, N. Mehrdad, L. Janani, and H. Shahsavari. "Leadership Identity Development Through Reflection and Feedback in

Team-Based Learning Medical Student Teams." Teaching and Learning in Medicine 30, no. 1 (2018): 76–83.

Fenning, Kristine. "Cohort Based Learning: Application to Learning Organizations and Student Academic Success." College Quarterly 7, no. 1 (2004): n1.

Goyal, M., S. Singh, E. M. Sibinga, N. F. Gould, A. Rowland-Seymour, R. Sharma, Z. Berger, D. Sleicher, D. D. Maron, H. M. Shihab, P. D. Ranasinghe, S. Linn, S. Saha, E. B. Bass, and J. A. Haythornthwaite. "Meditation programs for psychological stress and well-being: a systematic review and meta-analysis." JAMA Internal Medicine 174, no. 3 (2014): 357–68. *https://doi.org/10.1001/jamainternmed.2013.13018.*

Tang, Y. Y., B. K. Hölzel, and M. I. Posner. "The neuroscience of mindfulness meditation." Nature Reviews Neuroscience 16, no. 4 (2015): 213–25. *https://doi.org/10.1038/nrn3916.*

Chapter 5

Santidhammo Bhikkhu. "Maha Ghosananda: The Buddha of the Battlefield." S.R. Printing, 2009.

Michl, Louisa C., Katie A. McLaughlin, Kathrine Shepherd, and Susan Nolen-Hokesema. "Rumination as a Mechanism Linking Stressful Life Events to Symptoms of Depression and Anxiety: Longitudinal Evidence in Early Adolescents and Adults." Journal of Abnormal Psychology 122, no. 2 (2013): 339–52.

Bonnet, Michael H. and Donna L. Arand. "Evaluation and Diagnosis of Insomnia in Adults." In UpToDate, edited by Ruth Benca and April F. Eichler. Wolters Kluwer, October 4, 2022. *https://www.uptodate.com/contents/evaluation-and-diagnosis-of-insomnia-in-adults.*

"Know Your Brain: Default Mode Network." Neuroscientifically Challenged, accessed May 2, 2023. *https://neuroscientifically-challenged.com/posts/know-your-brain-default-mode-network.*

Posner, Jonathan, Christine Park, and Zhishun Wang. "Connecting the Dots: A Review of Resting Connectivity MRI Studies in Attention-Deficit/Hyperactivity Disorder." Neuropsychology Review 24, no. 1 (2014): 3–15.

Liu, C., Y. Liu , Y. Xin, and Y. Wang. "Circadian secretion rhythm of GLP-1 and its influencing factors." Frontiers in Endocrinology 13 (2022): 991397. *https://doi.org/10.3389/fendo.2022.991397.*

Maffei, Massimo E. "5-Hydroxytryptophan (5-HTP): Natural Occurrence, Analysis, Biosynthesis, Biotechnology, Physiology and Toxicology." International Journal of Molecular Sciences 22, no. 1 (2020): 181.

Reddy, Sujana, Vamsi Reddy, and Sandeep Sharma. "Physiology, Circadian Rhythm." In StatPearls. Treasure Island (FL): StatPearls Publishing, May 8, 2022. *https://www.ncbi.nlm.nih.gov/books/NBK519507/.*

Liu, Jiabei, Shannon J. Clough, Anthony J. Hutchinson, Ekue B. Adamah-Biassi, Marina Popovska-Gorevski, and Margarita L. Dubocovich. "MT1 and MT2 Melatonin Receptors: A Therapeutic Perspective." Annual Review of Pharmacology and Toxicology 56 (2016): 361–83.

Trauer, James M., Mary Y. Qian, Joseph S. Boyle, and Shantha M. W. Rajaratnam. "Cognitive Behavioral Therapy for Chronic Insomnia: A Systematic Review and Meta-Analysis." Annals of Internal Medicine 163, no. 3 (2015): 191–204.

Chapter 6

Gnocchi, Davide and Giovannella Bruscalupi. "Circadian Rhythms and Hormonal Homeostasis: Pathophysiological Implications." Biology 6, no. 1 (2017): 10.

"Vitamin D: Fact Sheet for Health Professionals." National Institutes of Health—Office of Dietary Supplements, updated August 12, 2022. *https://ods.od.nih.gov/factsheets/VitaminD-HealthProfessional/.*

Anjum, Ibrar, Syeda S. Jaffery, Muniba Fayyaz, Zarak Samoo, and Sheraz Anjum. "The Role of Vitamin D in Brain Health: A Mini Literature Review." Cureus 10, no. 7 (2018): e2960.

Khoshbakht, Yadollah, Reza Bidaki, and Amin Salehi-Abargouei. "Vitamin D Status and Attention Deficit Hyperactivity Disorder: A Systematic Review and Meta-Analysis of Observational Studies." Advances in Nutrition 9, no. 1 (2018): 9–20.

Zajac, Ian T., Mary Barnes, Paul Cavuoto, Gary Wittert, and Manny Noakes. "The Effects of Vitamin D-Enriched Mushrooms and Vitamin D3 on Cognitive Performance and Mood in Healthy Elderly Adults: A Randomised, Double-Blinded, Placebo-Controlled Trial." Nutrients 12, no. 12 (2020): 3847.

Abboud, Myriam. "Vitamin D Supplementation and Sleep: A Systematic Review and Meta-Analysis of Intervention Studies." Nutrients 14, no. 5 (2022): 1076.

Shieh, Albert, Rene F. Chun, Christina Ma, Sten Witzel, Briana Meyer, Brandon Rafison, Leon Swinkels, Tonnie Huijs, Sam Pepkowitz, and Brett Holmquist. "Effects of High-Dose Vitamin D2 Versus D3 on Total and Free 25-Hydroxyvitamin D and Markers of Calcium Balance." The Journal of Clinical Endocrinology and Metabolism 101, no. 8 (2016): 3070–8. *https://doi.org/10.1210/jc.2016-1871.*

Weiss, Roy E., M. A. Stein, B. Trommer, and S. Refetoff. "Attention-Deficit Hyperactivity Disorder and Thyroid Function." The Journal of Pediatrics 123, no. 4 (1993): 539–45.

Green, Max E., Victor Bernet, and Joseph Cheung. "Thyroid Dysfunction and Sleep Disorders." Frontiers in Endocrinology 12 (2021): 725829.

Dhillon-Smith, R. K., A. Tobias, P. P. Smith, L. J. Middleton, K. K. Sunner, K. Baker, S. Farrell-Carver, R. Bender-Atik, R. Agrawal, K. Bhatia, et al. "The Prevalence of Thyroid Dysfunction and Autoimmunity in Women With History of Miscarriage or Subfertility." J Clin Endocrinol Metab, 105(8): dgaa302. DOI: 10.1210/clinem/dgaa302.

Chapter 7

Kleinridders, Andre, Weikang Cai, Laura Cappellucci, Armen Ghazarian, Williams R. Collins, Sara G. Vienberg, Emmanuel N. Pothos, and C. Ronald Kahn. "Insulin Resistance in Brain Alters Dopamine Turnover and Causes Behavioral Disorders." Proceedings of the National Academy of Sciences 112.10 (2015): 10.1073/pnas.1500877112.

Won, Eunsoo, and Yong-Ku Kim. "Neuroinflammation-Associated Alterations of the Brain as Potential Neural Bio-markers in Anxiety Disorders." International Journal of Molecular Sciences 21, no. 18 (2020): 6546.

da Silva, Luiz Augusto, Leandro de Freitas, Thiago Emannuel Medeiros, Raul Osiecki, Renan Garcia Michel, André Luiz Snak, and Carlos Malfatti. "Caffeine Modifies Blood Glucose Availability During Prolonged Low-Intensity Exercise in Individuals With Type-2 Diabetes." Colombia Medica 45 (2) (2014): 72–76. *https://doi.org/10.25100/cm.v45i2.1477.*

Zaharieva, D. P., L. A. Miadovnik, C. P. Rowan, et al. "Effects of acute caffeine supplementation on reducing exercise-associated hypoglycaemia in individuals with Type 1 diabetes mellitus." Diabetic Medicine 33, no. 4 (2016): 488–96. DOI: 10.1111/dme.12857.

Alasmari, F. "Caffeine induces neurobehavioral effects through modulating neurotransmitters." Saudi Pharmaceutical Journal 28, no. 4 (2020): 445–51. DOI: 10.1016/j.jsps.2020.02.005.

Quinlan, P., J. Lane, and L. Aspinall. "Effects of hot tea, coffee and water ingestion on physiological responses and mood: the role of caffeine, water and beverage type." Psychopharmacology (Berl) 134, no. 2 (1997): 164–73. DOI: 10.1007/s002130050438.

Pandolfo, P., N. J. Machado, A. Köfalvi, R. N. Takahashi, and R. A. Cunha. "Caffeine regulates frontocorticostriatal dopamine transporter density and improves attention and cognitive deficits in an animal model of attention deficit hyperactivity disorder." European Neuropsychopharmacology 23, no. 4 (2013): 317–28. DOI: 10.1016/j.euroneuro.2012.04.011.

van Dam, R. M., W. J. Pasman, and P. Verhoef. "Effects of Coffee Consumption on Fasting Blood Glucose and Insulin Concentrations: Randomized controlled trials in healthy volunteers." Diabetes Care 27, no. 12 (2004): 2990–2. *https://doi.org/10.2337/diacare.27.12.2990.*

Ferreira, D. D., B. Stutz, F. G. de Mello, R. A. M. Reis, and R. C. C. Kubrusly. "Caffeine potentiates the release of GABA mediated by NMDA receptor activation: Involvement of A1 adenosine receptors." Neuroscience 281C (2014): 208–15.

Adan, A., and J. M. Serra-Grabulosa. "Effects of caffeine and glucose, alone and combined, on cognitive performance." Human Psychopharmacology 25, no. 4 (2010): 310–7.

Koppelstaetter, F., T. D. Poeppel, C. M. Siedentopf, et al. "Does caffeine modulate verbal working memory processes? An fMRI study." Neuroimage 39, no. 1 (2008): 492–9.

Liguori, A., J. R. Hughes, and J. A. Grass. "Absorption and

subjective effects of caffeine from coffee, cola and capsules." Pharmacology, Biochemistry, and Behavior 58, no. 3 (1997): 721–6.

Scholey, A. B., and D. O. Kennedy. "Cognitive and physiological effects of an 'energy drink': an evaluation of the whole drink and of glucose, caffeine and herbal flavoring fractions." Psychopharmacology 176, no. 3-4 (2004): 320–30. *https://doi.org/10.1007/s00213-004-1935-2.*

Serra-Grabulosa, J. M., A. Adan, C. Falcón, and N. Bargalló. "Glucose and caffeine effects on sustained attention: an exploratory fMRI study." Human Psychopharmacology 25, no. 7-8 (2010): 543–52.

Smit, H. J., and P. J. Rogers. "Effects of low doses of caffeine on cognitive performance, mood and thirst in low and higher caffeine consumers." Psychopharmacology (Berl) 152, no. 2 (2000): 167–73.

Urquiza, Sandra P., and Michelle L. Vieyra. "Assessing the Synergistic Effect of Caffeine and Sugar on Cognitive Performance in Undergraduate Students." Journal of the South Carolina Academy of Science 13 (2015): 6.

Hill, D., M. Conner, F. Clancy, R. Moss, S. Wilding, M. Bristow, and D. B. O'Connor. "Stress and eating behaviours in healthy adults: a systematic review and meta-analysis." Health Psychology Review 16, no. 2 (2022): 280–304. *https://doi.org/10.1080/17437199.2021.1923406.*

Chapter 8

Simopoulos, Artemis P. "The Importance of the Ratio of Omega-6/Omega-3 Essential Fatty Acids." Biomedicine & Pharmacotherapy 56, no. 8 (2002): 365–79.

Simopoulos, Artemis P. "Omega-3 Fatty Acids in Inflammation and Autoimmune Diseases." Journal of the American College of Nutrition 21, no. 6 (2002): 495–505.

Agostoni C., M. Nobile, V. Ciappolino, G. Delvecchio, A. Tesei, S. Turolo, A. Crippa, A. Mazzocchi, C. A. Altamura, and P. Brambilla. "The Role of Omega-3 Fatty Acids in Developmental Psychopathology: A Systematic Review on Early Psychosis, Autism, and ADHD." International Journal of Molecular Sciences 18, no. 12 (2017): 2608.

Derbyshire, Emma. "Brain Health across the Lifespan: A Systematic Review on the Role of Omega-3 Fatty Acid Supplements." Nutrients 10, no. 8 (2018): 1094.

Deane, Katherine H. O., et al. "Omega-3 and Polyunsaturated Fat for Prevention of Depression and Anxiety Symptoms: Systematic Review and Meta-Analysis of Randomised Trials." The British Journal of Psychiatry: The Journal of Mental Science 218, no. 3 (2021): 135–42.

Tandon, Anushree, Puneet Kaur, Amandeep Dhir, and Matti Mäntymäki. "Sleepless due to social media? Investigating problematic sleep due to social media and social media sleep hygiene." Computers in Human Behavior 113 (2020): 106487. DOI: 10.1016/j.chb.2020.106487.

Bourre, Jean-Marie. "Roles of Unsaturated Fatty Acids (Especially Omega-3 Fatty Acids) in the Brain at Various Ages and during Ageing." The Journal of Nutrition, Health & Aging 8, no. 3 (2004): 163–74.

Chapter 9

Taitelbaum-Swead, R., Z. Kozol, and L. Fostick. "Listening Effort Among Adults With and Without Attention-Deficit/ Hyperactivity Disorder." Journal of Speech, Language, and Hearing Research: JSLHR 62, no. 12 (2019): 4554–63. *https://doi.org/10.1044/2019_JSLHR-H-19-0134*.

Volkow, N. D., and J. M. Swanson. "Clinical practice: Adult attention deficit-hyperactivity disorder." The New England Journal of Medicine 369, no. 20 (2013): 1935–44. DOI: 10.1056/NEJMcp1212625.

Cross-Villasana, F., K. Finke, K. Hennig-Fast, B. Kilian, I. Wiegand, H. J. Müller, H. J. Möller, and T. Töllner. "The Speed of Visual Attention and Motor-Response Decisions in Adult Attention-Deficit/Hyperactivity Disorder." Biological Psychiatry 78, no. 2 (2015): 107–15. *https://doi.org/10.1016/j.biopsych.2015.01.016*.

Bekker, E. M., C. C. E. Overtoom, J. J. S. Kooij, J. K. Buitelaar, M. N. Verbaten, and J. L. Kenemans. "Disentangling deficits in adults with attention-deficit/hyperactivity disorder." Archives of General Psychiatry 62, no. 10 (2005): 1129–36. *https://doi.org/10.1001/archpsyc.62.10.1129*.

Doyle, A. E. "Executive functions in attention-deficit/ hyperactivity disorder." The Journal of Clinical Psychiatry 67 Suppl 8 (2006): 21–6.

Agnew-Blais, J. C., G. V. Polanczyk, A. Danese, J. Wertz, T. E. Moffitt, and L. Arseneault. "Evaluation of the Persistence, Remission, and Emergence of Attention-Deficit/Hyperactivity Disorder in Young Adulthood." JAMA Psychiatry 73, no. 7 (2016): 713–20. DOI: 10.1001/jamapsychiatry.2016.0465.

Small, G. W., J. Lee, A. Kaufman, J. Jalil, P. Siddarth, H. Gaddipati, T. D. Moody, and S. Y. Bookheimer. "Brain health consequences of digital technology use." Dialogues in Clinical Neuroscience 22, no. 2 (2020): 179–87. https://doi.org/10.31887/ DCNS.2020.22.2/gsmall.

Beyens, Ine, Patti M. Valkenburg, and Jessica Taylor Piotrowski. "Screen media use and ADHD-related behaviors: Four decades of research." Proceedings of the National Academy of Sciences 115, no. 40 (2018): 9875–81. Accessed October 1, 2018. https://doi.org/10.1073/pnas.1611611114.

Young, S., N. Adamo, B. B. Ásgeirsdóttir, P. Branney, M. Beckett, W. Colley, S. Cubbin, Q. Deeley, E. Farrag, G. Gudjonsson, et al. "Females with ADHD: An expert consensus statement taking a lifespan approach providing guidance for the identification and treatment of attention-deficit/hyperactivity disorder in girls and women." BMC Psychiatry 20, no. 1 (2020): 404. DOI: 10.1186/s12888-020-02707-9.

Draheim, C., R. Pak, A. A. Draheim, and R. W. Engle. "The role of attention control in complex real-world tasks."

Psychonomic Bulletin & Review 29, no. 4 (2022): 1143–97. DOI: 10.3758/s13423-021-02052-2.

Lorenz-Spreen, P., B. M. Mønsted, P. Hövel, and S. Lehman. "Accelerating dynamics of collective attention." Nature Communications 10 (2019): 1759. https://doi.org/10.1038/s41467-019-09311-w.

Torgersen, T., B. Gjervan, M. B. Lensing, and K. Rasmussen. "Optimal management of ADHD in older adults." Neuropsychiatric Disease and Treatment 12 (2016): 79–87. https://doi.org/10.2147/NDT.S59271.

Mitchell, J. T., E. M. McIntyre, J. S. English, M. F. Dennis, J. C. Beckham, and S. H. Kollins. "A Pilot Trial of Mindfulness Meditation Training for ADHD in Adulthood: Impact on Core Symptoms, Executive Functioning, and Emotion Dysregulation." Journal of Attention Disorders 21, no. 13 (2017): 1105–20. https://doi.org/10.1177/1087054713513328.

Guntuku, S. C., J. R. Ramsay, R. M. Merchant, and L. H. Ungar. "Language of ADHD in Adults on Social Media." Journal of Attention Disorders 23, no. 12 (2019): 1475–85. https://doi.org/10.1177/1087054717738083.

Asherson, P., R. Akehurst, J. J. Sandro. Kooij, M. Huss, M., K. Beusterien, R. Sasané, S. Gholizadeh, and Hodgkins, P. (2012). "Under diagnosis of adult ADHD: Cultural influences and societal burden." Journal of Attention Disorders 16 (Suppl. 5) (2012): 20S–38S.

Chamberlain, S. R., K. Ioannidis, E. W. Leppink, F. Niaz,

S. A. Redden, and J. E. Grant. "ADHD symptoms in non-treatment seeking young adults: Relationship with other forms of impulsivity." CNS Spectrums, 22 (2017): 22–30.

Miklósi, M., O. Máté, K. Somogyi, and M. Szabó. (2016). "Adult attention deficit hyperactivity disorder symptoms, perceived stress, and well-being". The Journal of Nervous and Mental Disease, 204 (2016): 364–9.

Ramsay, J. R. "Assessment and monitoring of treatment response in adult ADHD patients: Current perspectives." Neuropsychiatric Disease and Treatment, 13 (2017): 221–32.

Settanni, M., D. Marengo, M. A. Fabris, and C. Longobardi. "The Interplay Between ADHD Symptoms and Time Perspective in Addictive Social Media Use: A Study on Adolescent Facebook Users." Children and Youth Services Review 89 (2018): 165–70. https://doi.org/10.1016/j.childyouth.2018.04.031.

Panagiotidi, M. "Problematic Video Game Play and ADHD Traits in an Adult Population." Cyberpsychology, Behavior, and Social Networking, May 2017, 292–5. http://doi.org/10.1089/cyber.2016.0676.

Fayyad, J., R. De Graaf, R. Kessler, et al. "Cross-National Prevalence and Correlates of Adult Attention-Deficit Hyperactivity Disorder." British Journal of Psychiatry, 190 (2007): 402.

Yeung, A., E. Ng, and E. Abi-Jaoude. "TikTok and Attention-Deficit/Hyperactivity Disorder: A Cross-Sectional Study of

Social Media Content Quality." Canadian Journal of Psychiatry, 67(12) (2022): 899–906. DOI: 10.1177/07067437221082854.

Aly, M., and N. B. Turk-Browne. "How Hippocampal Memory Shapes, and Is Shaped By, Attention." In D. E. Hannula & M. C. Duff (Eds.), The Hippocampus from Cells to Systems (2017): 369–403. Cham: Springer.

Faraone, S. V., J. Biederman, and E. Mick. "The age-dependent decline of attention deficit hyperactivity disorder: A meta-analysis of follow-up studies." Psychological Medicine, 36(2) (2006): 159–65.

Chapter 10

Smith, Kyle S., and Ann M. Graybiel. "Investigating habits: Strategies, technologies and models." Frontiers in Behavioral Neuroscience, 8 (2014): 78680. *https://doi.org/10.3389/fnbeh.2014.00039.*

Fogg, BJ. "A behavior model for persuasive design." In Proceedings of the 4th International Conference on Persuasive Technology (Persuasive '09) (2009): 1–7. New York: ACM. *https://doi.org/10.1145/1541948.1541999.*

Clear, James. *Atomic Habits.* New York, New York: Avery, an imprint of Penguin Random House, 2018.

Clear, James. "How long does it take to form a new habit? (Backed by science)." James Clear's website, *https://jamesclear.com/new-habit.*

Fogg, BJ. "Tiny Habits: The Small Changes That Change Everything." Boston, MA: Houghton Mifflin Harcourt, 2019.

Neal, D. T., W. Wood, and A. Drolet. "How do people adhere to goals when willpower is low? The profits (and pitfalls) of strong habits." Journal of Personality and Social Psychology, 104(6) (2013): 959.

"Defense Mechanisms: Theoretical, Research and Clinical Perspectives." Edited by Uwe Hentschel, Gudmund Smith, Juris G. Draguns, and Wolfram Ehlers. Elsevier, 2004.

Blanco, Carlos, Leonie Kampe, Melanie M. Wall, Shang-Min Liu, Eve Caligor, and Mark Olfson. "Approximating defense mechanisms in a national study of adults: prevalence and correlates with functioning." Translational Psychiatry, 13(1) (2023): 21. DOI: 10.1038/s41398-022-02303-3.

Chapter 11

Liu J., S. J. Clough, A. J. Hutchinson, E. B. Adamah-Biassi, M. Popovska-Gorevski, and M. L. Dubocovich. "MT1 and MT2 Melatonin Receptors: A Therapeutic Perspective." Annual Review of Pharmacology and Toxicology 56 (2016): 361–83.

Choi, K., Y. J. Lee, S. Park, N. K. Je, and H. S. Suh. "Efficacy of Melatonin for Chronic Insomnia: Systematic Reviews and Meta-Analyses." Sleep Medicine Reviews 66 (2022): 101692. https://doi.org/10.1016/j.smrv.2022.101692.

Schroeck, J. L., J. Ford, E. L. Conway, K. E. Kurtzhalts,

M. E. Gee, K. A. Vollmer, and K. A. Mergenhagen. "Review of Safety and Efficacy of Sleep Medicines in Older Adults." Clinical Therapeutics 38, no. 11 (2016): 2340–72. https://doi.org/10.1016/j.clinthera.2016.09.010.

Minich, D. M., M. Henning, C. Darley, M. Fahoum, C. B. Schuler, and J. Frame. "Is Melatonin the 'Next Vitamin D'?: A Review of Emerging Science, Clinical Uses, Safety, and Dietary Supplements." Nutrients 14, no. 19 (2022): 3934. https://doi.org/10.3390/nu14193934.

Smolensky, M. H., L. L. Sackett-Lundeen, and F. Portaluppi. "Nocturnal Light Pollution and Underexposure to Daytime Sunlight: Complementary Mechanisms of Circadian Disruption and Related Diseases." Chronobiology International 32, no. 8 (2015): 1029–48. https://doi.org/10.3109/07420528.2015.1072002.

Richardson, G., and B. Tate. "Hormonal and Pharmacological Manipulation of the Circadian Clock: Recent Developments and Future Strategies." Sleep 23 Suppl 3 (2000): S77–S85.

Touitou, Y., A. Reinberg, and D. Touitou. "Association between Light at Night, Melatonin Secretion, Sleep Deprivation, and the Internal Clock: Health Impacts and Mechanisms of Circadian Disruption." Life Sciences 173 (2017): 94–106. https://doi.org/10.1016/j.lfs.2017.02.008.

Liu, C., Y. Liu, Y. Xin, and Y. Wang. "Circadian Secretion Rhythm of GLP-1 and Its Influencing Factors." Frontiers in Endocrinology 13 (2022): 991397. https://doi.org/10.3389/fendo.2022.991397.

Benedict, C. "Melatonin's Potential Side Effects: It May Be in Your Genes." Mayo Clinic Proceedings 97, no. 7 (2022): 1401. *https://doi.org/10.1016/j.mayocp.2022.05.011.*

Gamble, K. L., R. Berry, S. J. Frank, and M. E. Young. "Circadian Clock Control of Endocrine Factors." Nature Reviews. Endocrinology 10, no. 8 (2014): 466–75. *https://doi.org/10.1038/nrendo.2014.78.*

Arab, A., N. Rafie, R. Amani, et al. "The Role of Magnesium in Sleep Health: A Systematic Review of Available Literature." Biological Trace Element Research 201 (2023): 121–28. *https://doi.org/10.1007/s12011-022-03162-1.*

Zhang, Yijia, et al. "Association of Magnesium Intake with Sleep Duration and Sleep Quality: Findings from the CARDIA Study." Sleep 45, no. 4 (2022): zsab276. *https://doi.org/10.1093/sleep/zsab276.*

Ates, M., S. Kizildag, O. Yuksel, et al. "Dose-Dependent Absorption Profile of Different Magnesium Compounds." Biological Trace Element Research 192, no. 2 (2019): 244–51. *https://doi.org/10.1007/s12011-019-01663-0.*

Abbasi, B., M. Kimiagar, K. Sadeghniiat, M. M. Shirazi, M. Hedayati, and B. Rashidkhani. "The Effect of Magnesium Supplementation on Primary Insomnia in Elderly: A Double-Blind Placebo-Controlled Clinical Trial." Journal of Research in Medical Sciences 17, no. 12 (2012): 1161–9. PMID: 23853635.

Morris, M. E. "Brain and CSF Magnesium Concentrations

during Magnesium Deficit in Animals and Humans: Neurological Symptoms." Magnesium Research 5 (1992): 303–13.

Ford, E. S., and A. H. Mokdad. "Dietary Magnesium Intake in a National Sample of US Adults." Journal of Nutrition 133 (2003): 2879–82.

Takase, Bonpei, et al. "Effect of Chronic Stress and Sleep Deprivation on Both Flow-Mediated Dilation in the Brachial Artery and the Intracellular Magnesium Level in Humans." Clinical Cardiology 27, no. 4 (2004): 223–7. DOI: 10.1002/clc.4960270411.

Maffei, Massimo E. "5-Hydroxytryptophan (5-HTP): Natural Occurrence, Analysis, Biosynthesis, Biotechnology, Physiology and Toxicology." International Journal of Molecular Sciences 22, no. 1 (2020): 181.

Birdsall, T. C. "5-Hydroxytryptophan: A Clinically-Effective Serotonin Precursor." Alternative Medicine Review 3, no. 4 (1998): 271–80.

Meloni, M., et al. "Preliminary Finding of a Randomized, Double-Blind, Placebo-Controlled, Crossover Study to Evaluate the Safety and Efficacy of 5-Hydroxytryptophan on REM Sleep Behavior Disorder in Parkinson's Disease." Sleep & Breathing = Schlaf & Atmung 26, no. 3 (2022): 1023–31. DOI: 10.1007/s11325-021-02417-w.

Rios, Patricia, Roberta Cardoso, Deanna Morra, Vera Nincic, Zahra Goodarzi, Bechara Farah, Sharada Harricharan, et al. "Comparative Effectiveness and Safety of Pharmacological and Non-Pharmacological Interventions for Insomnia: An Overview of Reviews." Systematic Reviews 8, no. 1 (2019): 281. *https://doi.org/10.1186/s13643-019-1163-9.*

Parrino, Liborio, Peter Halasz, Anna Szucs, Robert J. Thomas, Nicoletta Azzi, Federica Rausa, Silvia Pizzarotti, et al. "Sleep Medicine: Practice, Challenges and New Frontiers." Frontiers in Neurology 13 (2022): 966659. *https://doi.org/10.3389/fneur.2022.966659.*

Gradisar, Michael, Amy R. Wolfson, Allison G. Harvey, Lauren Hale, Russell Rosenberg, and Charles A. Czeisler. "The Sleep and Technology Use of Americans: Findings from the National Sleep Foundation's 2011 Sleep in America Poll." Journal of Clinical Sleep Medicine 9, no. 12 (2013): 1291–9.

AlShareef, Saad M. "The Impact of Bedtime Technology Use on Sleep Quality and Excessive Daytime Sleepiness in Adults." Sleep Science 15, no. Spec 2 (2022): 318–27. DOI: 10.5935/1984-0063.20200128.

Liu, Min, and Jianghong Luo. "Relationship between Peripheral Blood Dopamine Level and Internet Addiction Disorder in Adolescents: A Pilot Study." International Journal of Clinical and Experimental Medicine 8 (2015): 9943–8.

Ayano, Getinet. "Dopamine: Receptors, Functions, Synthesis, Pathways, Locations and Mental Disorders: Review of Literatures." Journal of Mental Disorders and Treatment 2 (2016): 120. DOI: 10.4172/2471-271X.1000120.

Wise, Roy A. "Addictive Drugs and Brain Stimulation Reward." Annual Review of Neuroscience 19 (1996): 319–40.

Le Moal, Michel, and Hélène Simon. "Mesocorticolimbic Dopaminergic Network: Functional and Regulatory Roles." Physiological Reviews 71 (1991): 155–234.

Cook, Edwin H., Mark A. Stein, and Michael D. Krasowski, et al. "Association of Attention-Deficit Disorder and the Dopamine Transporter Gene." American Journal of Human Genetics 56 (1995): 993–8.

Chapter 12

Smolensky, Michael H., Linda L. Sackett-Lundeen, and Francesco Portaluppi. "Nocturnal Light Pollution and Underexposure to Daytime Sunlight: Complementary Mechanisms of Circadian Disruption and Related Diseases." Chronobiology International 32, no. 8 (2015): 1029–48. *https://doi.org/10.3109/07420528.2015.1072002.*

Richardson, G., and B. Tate. "Hormonal and Pharmacological Manipulation of the Circadian Clock: Recent Developments and Future Strategies." Sleep 23 Suppl 3 (2000): S77–S85.

Touitou, Y., A. Reinberg, and D. Touitou. "Association between Light at Night, Melatonin Secretion, Sleep Deprivation, and the Internal Clock: Health Impacts and Mechanisms of Circadian Disruption." Life Sciences 173 (2017): 94–106. *https://doi.org/10.1016/j.lfs.2017.02.008.*

Liu, C., Y. Liu, Y. Xin, and Y. Wang. "Circadian Secretion

Rhythm of GLP-1 and Its Influencing Factors." Frontiers in Endocrinology 13 (2022): 991397. *https://doi.org/10.3389/fendo.2022.991397.*

Al Kazhali, M., M. Shahwan, N. Hassan, and A. A. Jairoun. "Social Media Use Is Linked to Poor Sleep Quality: The Opportunities and Challenges to Support Evidence-Informed Policymaking in the UAE." Journal of Public Health 45, no. 1 (2023): 124–33. DOI: 10.1093/pubmed/fdab372.

Bhat, S., G. Pinto-Zipp, H. Upadhyay, and P. G. Polos. "'To Sleep, Perchance to Tweet': In-Bed Electronic Social Media Use and Its Associations with Insomnia, Daytime Sleepiness, Mood, and Sleep Duration in Adults." Sleep Health 4, no. 2 (2018): 166–73. DOI: 10.1016/j.sleh.2017.12.004.

Levenson, Jessica C., Ariel Shensa, Jaime E. Sidani, Jason B. Colditz, and Brian A. Primack. "The Association Between Social Media Use and Sleep Disturbance Among Young Adults." Preventive Medicine 85 (2016): 36–41. DOI:10.1016/j.ypmed.2016.01.001.

Orzech, Kathryn M., Michael A. Grandner, Brandy M. Roane, and Mary A. Carskadon. "Digital Media Use in the 2 h Before Bedtime Is Associated with Sleep Variables in University Students." Computers in Human Behavior 55, Part A (2016): 43–50. DOI: 10.1016/j.chb.2015.08.049.

Brown, T. M., G. C. Brainard, C. Cajochen, C. A. Czeisler, J. P. Hanifin, S. W. Lockley, R. J. Lucas, et al. "Recommendations for Daytime, Evening, and Nighttime Indoor Light Exposure to Best Support Physiology, Sleep, and Wakefulness in Healthy Adults." PLoS Biology 20, no. 3 (2022): e3001571. *https://doi.org/10.1371/journal.pbio.3001571.*

Lawrenson, J. G., C. C. Hull, and L. E. Downie. "The Effect of Blue-Light Blocking Spectacle Lenses on Visual Performance, Macular Health and the Sleep-Wake Cycle: A Systematic Review of the Literature." Ophthalmic & Physiological Optics 37, no. 6 (2017): 644–54. *https://doi.org/10.1111/opo.12406.*

Chang, A. M., D. Aeschbach, J. F. Duffy, and C. A. Czeisler. "Evening Use of Light-Emitting eReaders Negatively Affects Sleep, Circadian Timing, and Next-Morning Alertness." Proceedings of the National Academy of Sciences of the United States of America 112, no. 4 (2015): 1232–7. *https://doi.org/10.1073/pnas.1418490112.*

Cho, Y., S. H. Ryu, B. R. Lee, K. H. Kim, E. Lee, and J. Choi. "Effects of Artificial Light at Night on Human Health: A Literature Review of Observational and Experimental Studies Applied to Exposure Assessment." Chronobiology International 32, no. 9 (2015): 1294–310. *https://doi.org/10.3109/07420528.2015.1073158.*

Rios, P., et al. "Comparative Effectiveness and Safety of Pharmacological and Non-Pharmacological Interventions for Insomnia: An Overview of Reviews." Systematic Reviews 8, no. 1 (2019): 281. *https://doi.org/10.1186/s13643-019-1163-9.*

Parrino, L., et al. "Sleep Medicine: Practice, Challenges and New Frontiers." Frontiers in Neurology 13 (2022): 966659. *https://doi.org/10.3389/fneur.2022.966659.*

Tandon, Anushree, Puneet Kaur, Amandeep Dhir, and Matti Mäntymäki. "Sleepless due to social media? Investigating problematic sleep due to social media and social media sleep hygiene." Computers in Human Behavior 113 (2020): 106487. DOI: 10.1016/j.chb.2020.106487.

Scullin, M. K., et al. "The Effects of Bedtime Writing on Difficulty Falling Asleep: A Polysomnographic Study Comparing To-Do Lists and Completed Activity Lists." Journal of Experimental Psychology: General 147, no. 1 (2018): 139–46. DOI: 10.1037/xge0000374.

Chapter 13

Wehrenberg, Margaret. "Rumination: A Problem in Anxiety and Depression." Psychology Today, April 20, 2016. *https://www.psychologytoday.com/us/blog/depression-management-techniques/201604/rumination-a-problem-in-anxiety-and-depression.*

Hoyer, Jürgen, Andrew T. Gloster, and Philipp Yorck Herzberg. "Is Worry Different from Rumination? Yes, It Is More Predictive of Psychopathology!" GMS Psycho-Social-Medicine 6 (2009): Doc06.

Gustavson, Daniel E., et al. "Evidence for Transdiagnostic Repetitive Negative Thinking and Its Association with Rumination, Worry, and Depression and Anxiety Symptoms: A Commonality Analysis." Collabra Psychology 4, no. 1 (2018): 13.

Joubert, Amy E., et al. "Understanding the Experience of Rumination and Worry: A Descriptive Qualitative Survey

Study." The British Journal of Clinical Psychology 61, no. 4 (2022): 929.

Michl, Louisa C., et al. "Rumination as a Mechanism Linking Stressful Life Events to Symptoms of Depression and Anxiety: Longitudinal Evidence in Early Adolescents and Adults." Journal of Abnormal Psychology 122, no. 2 (2013): 339–52.

Valentino, M. "14 Proven Herbs, Nootropics, & Supplements to Crush Rumination & Enhance Mental Health." Valentino's Naturals, February 8, 2023. *https://valentinosnaturals.com/natural-supplements-rumination/.*

Karcı, Canan Kuygun, and Gonca Gül Celik. "Nutritional and Herbal Supplements in the Treatment of Obsessive Compulsive Disorder." General Psychiatry 33, no. 2 (2020): e100159.

Mallik, Adiel, and Frank A. Russo. "The Effects of Music & Auditory Beat Stimulation on Anxiety: A Randomized Clinical Trial." PLoS One 17, no. 3 (2022): e0259312.

Vinall, Marnie. "Can Shaking Help You Heal Stress and Trauma? Some Experts Say Yes." Healthline, March 5, 2021. *https://www.healthline.com/health/mental-health/can-shaking-your-body-heal-stress-and-trauma.*

Chenoweth, Hannah. "Binaural Beats Are Being Used as Sound Wave Therapy for Anxiety, but Does It Really Help?" Prevention, March 9, 2021. *https://www.prevention.com/health/mental-health/a35782370/binaural-beats-for-anxiety/.*

Thoma, Myriam V., et al. "The Effect of Music on the Human Stress Response." PLoS One 8, no. 8 (2013): e70156.

Lu, Guangli, et al. "Effects of Music Therapy on Anxiety: A Meta-Analysis of Randomized Controlled Trials." Psychiatry Research 304 (2021): 114137.

Chapter 14

Kleinridders, Andre, Weikang Cai, Laura Cappellucci, Armen Ghazarian, Will Collins, Sara Vienberg, Emmanuel Pothos, and C. Ronald Kahn. "Insulin Resistance in Brain Alters Dopamine Turnover and Causes Behavioral Disorders." Proceedings of the National Academy of Sciences 112, no. 11 (2015): 3463–8. *https://www.pnas.org/content/112/11/3463*.

Won, Eunsoo, and Yong-Ku Kim. "Neuroinflammation-Associated Alterations of the Brain as Potential Neural Biomarkers in Anxiety Disorders." International Journal of Molecular Sciences 21, no. 18 (2020): 6546. *https://www.mdpi. com/1422-0067/21/18/6546*.

Torres, Susan J. and Caryl A. Nowson. "Relationship between stress, eating behavior, and obesity." Nutrition (Burbank, Los Angeles County, Calif.) 23, no. 11–12 (2007): 887–94. *https:// doi.org/10.1016/j.nut.2007.08.008*.

Da Silva, Leonardo A., et al. "Caffeine modifies blood glucose availability during prolonged low-intensity exercise in individuals with type-2 diabetes." Colombian Medical (Cali) 45, no. 2 (2014): 72–6. *https://doi.org/10.25100/cm.v45i2.1477*.

Zaharieva, Despina P., et al. "Effects of acute caffeine supplementation on reducing exercise-associated hypoglycemia in individuals with Type 1 diabetes mellitus." Diabetic Medicine 33, no. 4 (2016): 488–96. DOI: 10.1111/dme.12857.

Alasmari, F. "Caffeine induces neurobehavioral effects through modulating neurotransmitters." Saudi Pharmaceutical Journal 28, no. 4 (2020): 445–51. DOI: 10.1016/j.jsps.2020.02.005.

Quinlan, P., J. Lane, and L. Aspinall. "Effects of hot tea, coffee and water ingestion on physiological responses and mood: the role of caffeine, water and beverage type." Psychopharmacology (Berl) 134, no. 2 (1997): 164–73. DOI: 10.1007/s002130050438. *https://pubmed.ncbi.nlm.nih.gov/9399380/*.

Pandolfo, P., N. J. Machado, A. Köfalvi, R. N. Takahashi, and R. A. Cunha. "Caffeine regulates frontocorticostriatal dopamine transporter density and improves attention and cognitive deficits in an animal model of attention deficit hyperactivity disorder." European Neuropsychopharmacology 23, no. 4 (2013): 317–28. DOI: 10.1016/j.euroneuro.2012.04.011. *https://pubmed.ncbi.nlm.nih.gov/22561003/*.

Van Dam, R. M., W. J. Pasman, and P. Verhoef. "Effects of Coffee Consumption on Fasting Blood Glucose and Insulin Concentrations: Randomized controlled trials in healthy volunteers." Diabetes Care 27, no. 12 (2004): 2990–2. *https://doi.org/10.2337/diacare.27.12.2990*.

Ferreira, D. D., B. Stutz, F. G. de Mello, R. A. Reis, and R. C. Kubrusly. "Caffeine potentiates the release of GABA mediated by NMDA receptor activation: Involvement of A1 adenosine receptors." Neuroscience 281C (2014): 208–15.

Adan, A. and J. M. Serra-Grabulosa. "Effects of caffeine and glucose, alone and combined, on cognitive performance." Hum Psychopharmacol 25, no. 4 (2010): 310–7.

Liguori, A., J. R. Hughes, and J. A. Grass. "Absorption and subjective effects of caffeine from coffee, cola and capsules." Pharmacology, Biochemistry, Behavior 58, no. 3 (1997): 721–6.

Quinlan, P., J. Lane, and L. Aspinall. "Effects of hot tea, coffee and water ingestion on physiological responses and mood: the role of caffeine, water and beverage type." Psychopharmacology (Berl) 134, no. 2 (1997): 164–73.

Scholey, A. B., and D. O. Kennedy. "Cognitive and physiological effects of an 'energy drink': an evaluation of the whole drink and of glucose, caffeine and herbal flavoring fractions." Psychopharmacology 176, no. 3-4 (2004): 320–30. *https://doi. org/10.1007/s00213-004-1935-2.*

Urquiza, Sandra P., and Michelle L. Vieyra. "Assessing the Synergistic Effect of Caffeine and Sugar on Cognitive Performance in Undergraduate Students." Journal of the South Carolina Academy of Science 13 (2015): 6.

Hill, D., M. Conner, F. Clancy, R. Moss, S. Wilding, M. Bristow, and D. B. O'Connor. "Stress and eating behaviours in healthy adults: a systematic review and meta-analysis." Health Psychology Review 16, no. 2 (2022): 280–304. *https://doi.org/ 10.1080/17437199.2021.1923406.*

Brenton-Peters, Jennifer, et al. "Self-compassion, Stress, and Eating Behaviour: Exploring the Effects of Self-compassion on

Dietary Choice and Food Craving After Laboratory-Induced Stress." International Journal of Behavioral Medicine 30, no. 3 (2023): 438–47. *https://doi.org/10.1007/s12529-022-10110-9.*

Chapter 15

Chianese, R., R. Coccurello, A. Viggiano, M. Scafuro, M. Fiore, G. Coppola, F. F. Operto, S. Fasano, S. Laye, R. Pierantoni, and R. Meccariello. "Impact of Dietary Fats on Brain Functions." Current Neuropharmacology 16, no. 7 (2018): 1059–85. *https://doi.org/10.2174/1570159X15666171017102547.*

Chang, Chia-Yu, Der-Shin Ke, and Jen-Yin Chen. "Essential fatty acids and human brain." Acta Neurol Taiwan 18, no. 4 (2009): 231–41. PMID: 20329590.

Fekete, Monika, et al. "Nutrition Strategies Promoting Healthy Aging: From Improvement of Cardiovascular and Brain Health to Prevention of Age-Associated Diseases." Nutrients 15, no. 1 (2022): 47. *https://doi.org/10.3390/nu15010047.*

Román, Gustavo C., et al. "Mediterranean diet: The role of long-chain ω-3 fatty acids in fish; polyphenols in fruits, vegetables, cereals, coffee, tea, cacao and wine; probiotics and vitamins in prevention of stroke, age-related cognitive decline, and Alzheimer disease." Revue neurologique 175, no. 10 (2019): 724–41.

Risérus, Ulf, Walter C. Willett, and Frank B. Hu. "Dietary fats and prevention of type 2 diabetes." Prog Lipid Res 48, no. 1 (2009): 44–51. *https://doi.org/10.1016/j.plipres.2008.10.002.*

Lichtenstein, Alice H., and Ursula S. Schwab. "Relationship of dietary fat to glucose metabolism." Atherosclerosis 150 (2000): 227–43.

Simopoulos, Artemis P. "The Importance of the Ratio of Omega-6/Omega-3 Essential Fatty Acids." Biomedicine & Pharmacotherapy 56, no. 8 (2002): 365–79.

Simopoulos, Artemis P. "Omega-3 Fatty Acids in Inflammation and Autoimmune Diseases." Journal of the American College of Nutrition 21, no. 6 (2002): 495–505.

Agostoni C, M. Nobile, V. Ciappolino, G. Delvecchio, A. Tesei, S. Turolo, A. Crippa, A. Mazzocchi, C. A. Altamura, and P. Brambilla. "The Role of Omega-3 Fatty Acids in Developmental Psychopathology: A Systematic Review on Early Psychosis, Autism, and ADHD." International Journal of Molecular Sciences 18, no. 12 (2017): 2608.

Derbyshire, Emma. "Brain Health across the Lifespan: A Systematic Review on the Role of Omega-3 Fatty Acid Supplements." Nutrients 10, no. 8 (2018): 1094.

Deane, Katherine H. O., et al. "Omega-3 and Polyunsaturated Fat for Prevention of Depression and Anxiety Symptoms: Systematic Review and Meta-Analysis of Randomised Trials." The British Journal of Psychiatry 218, no. 3 (2021): 135–42.

Tandon, Anushree, Puneet Kaur, Amandeep Dhir, and Matti Mäntymäki. "Sleepless due to social media? Investigating problematic sleep due to social media and social media sleep hygiene." Computers in Human Behavior 113 (2020):

106487. Accessed September 13, 2023. *https://doi.org/10.1016/j.chb.2020.106487.*

Bourre, Jean-Marie. "Roles of Unsaturated Fatty Acids (Especially Omega-3 Fatty Acids) in the Brain at Various Ages and during Ageing." The Journal of Nutrition, Health & Aging 8, no. 3 (2004): 163–74.

Imamura, Fumiaki, et al. "Effects of Saturated Fat, Polyunsaturated Fat, Monounsaturated Fat, and Carbohydrate on Glucose-Insulin Homeostasis: A Systematic Review and Meta-analysis of Randomised Controlled Feeding Trials." PLoS Medicine 13, no. 7 (2016): e1002087. *https://doi.org/10.1371/journal.pmed.1002087.*

Chapter 16

"Vitamin D: Fact Sheet for Health Professionals." National Institutes of Health—Office of Dietary Supplements. Updated August 12, 2022. *https://ods.od.nih.gov/factsheets/VitaminD-HealthProfessional/.*

Anjum, Ibrar, Syeda S. Jaffrey, Muniba Fayyaz, Zarak Samoo, and Sheraz Anjum. "The Role of Vitamin D in Brain Health: A Mini Literature Review." Cureus 10, no. 7 (2018): e2960.

Khoshbakht, Yadollah, Reza Bidaki, and Amin Salehi-Abargouei. "Vitamin D Status and Attention Deficit Hyperactivity Disorder: A Systematic Review and Meta-Analysis of Observational Studies." Advances in Nutrition 9, no. 1 (2018): 9–20.

Zajac, Ian T., Mary Barnes, Paul Cavuoto, Gary Wittert, and Manny Noakes. "The Effects of Vitamin D-Enriched Mushrooms and Vitamin D3 on Cognitive Performance and Mood in Healthy Elderly Adults: A Randomised, Double-Blinded, Placebo-Controlled Trial." Nutrients 12, no. 12 (2020): 3847.

Abboud, Myriam. "Vitamin D Supplementation and Sleep: A Systematic Review and Meta-Analysis of Intervention Studies." Nutrients 14, no. 5 (2022): 1076.

Shieh, Albert, Rene F. Chun, Christina Ma, Sten Witzel, Briana Meyer, Brandon Rafison, Leon Swinkels, Tonnie Huijs, Sam Pepkowitz, and Brett Holmquist. "Effects of High-Dose Vitamin D2 Versus D3 on Total and Free 25-Hydroxyvitamin D and Markers of Calcium Balance." The Journal of Clinical Endocrinology and Metabolism 101, no. 8 (2016): 3070–8.

Weiss, Roy E., M. A. Stein, B. Trommer, and S. Refetoff. "Attention-Deficit Hyperactivity Disorder and Thyroid Function." The Journal of Pediatrics 123, no. 4 (1993): 539–45.

Green, Max E., Victor Bernet, and Joseph Cheung. "Thyroid Dysfunction and Sleep Disorders." Frontiers in Endocrinology 12 (2021): 725829.

Dhillon-Smith, R. K., A. Tobias, P. P. Smith, L. J. Middleton, K. K. Sunner, K. Baker, S. Farrell-Carver, R. Bender-Atik, R. Agrawal, K. Bhatia, et al. "The Prevalence of Thyroid Dysfunction and Autoimmunity in Women with History of Miscarriage or Subfertility." The Journal of Clinical Endocrinology & Metabolism (2020). DOI: 10.1210/clinem/dgaa302.

Wiegand, A., M. H. J. Munk, S. Drohm, A. J. Fallgatter, J. L. MacIsaac, M. S. Kobor, V. Nieratschker, and B. Kreifelts. "Neural correlates of attentional control in social anxiety disorder: the impact of early-life adversity and DNA methylation." J Psychiatry Neurosci. 2021 Dec 16;46(6): E663–E674. DOI: 10.1503/jpn.210064.

Binder, E. B. "The role of FKBP5, a co-chaperone of the glucocorticoid receptor in the pathogenesis and therapy of affective and anxiety disorders." Psychoneuroendocrinology 34(Suppl 1): S186–195. (2009).

Glad, Camilla A. M., et al. "Reduced DNA methylation and psychopathology following endogenous hypercortisolism— a genome-wide study." Scientific Reports 7 (2017): 44445. DOI: 10.1038/srep44445.

Hing, B., C. Gardner, and J. B. Potash. "Effects of negative stressors on DNA methylation in the brain: implications for mood and anxiety disorders." American Journal of Medicine Genetics. Part B, Neuropsychiatric genetics. 2014 Oct;165B(7): 541–54. DOI: 10.1002/ajmg.b.32265. Epub 2014 Aug 19. PMID: 25139739.

Miriam A Schiele, Michael G Gottschalk, Katharina Domschke. "The applied implications of epigenetics in anxiety, affective and stress-related disorders—A review and synthesis on psychosocial stress, psychotherapy and prevention." Clinical Psychology Review 77 (2020): 101830. https://doi. org/10.1016/j.cpr.2020.101830.

Bjelland, Ingvar, et al. "Folate, Vitamin B12, Homocysteine, and the MTHFR 677C→T Polymorphism in Anxiety and Depression: The Hordaland Homocysteine Study." Archives of Gen Psychiatry. 2003;60(6):618–26. DOI: 10.1001/archpsyc.60.6.618.

ACKNOWLEDGMENTS

"To know that even one life has breathed easier because you have lived. This is to have succeeded."

—Ralph Waldo Emerson

Storytellers raised me, and I became the vessel to receive stories in that process. It is a gift that helped me as a doctor and today as an award-winning speaker, female founder, and Chief Wellness Officer. I start by thanking anyone who has opened their heart to share their stories with me, starting with my elders, friends, colleagues, epilepsy patients, executive coaching clients, neighbors in our condo building, other dog parents meeting Rahja and me on the street, random passengers on my Delta Air Lines flights, and our associates at Evolution Hospitality, where I am the Chief Wellness Officer, or officially "Our Homie Dr. Romie."

The Busy Brain Cure was written for the thousands of people who stopped me after my speaking engagements to share their stories of how stress, burnout, and Busy Brain symptoms impacted their lives. I want to especially acknowledge those of you who opened your hearts and allowed me to write your stories in this book so that others may heal.

Every time I attempted the acknowledgment section of this book, I would start to sob so deeply where I would choke on salty tears and blow out my nose into gobs of paper towels. Delicate tissues failed as I comforted myself by stepping away from my MacBook Pro. Then Eden from the incredible team at Hanover Square Press emailed me during manuscript edits asking for this section of the book. I feared I would forget to thank someone, and thinking of my acknowledgments unlocked my unprocessed grief.

There are many people I want to thank who are no longer on Mother Earth with us. I hope I said at least one heartfelt thank-you while you were still alive. If you are reading this, take a brainPAUSE and say "I love you" to all who have helped you breathe easier in this lifetime. Nanni, Mrs. Georgia Reed, Aunty Nosheen, Papa Cunningham, Aunty Zenith, Aunty Hina, Aunty Shaista, and so many of my Aunties, who were my teachers, mentors, and prayer holders, I send a prayer of love and gratitude up to you in Heaven. I felt your Divine presence when I would wake up at 3:33 a.m. out of bed with a heart full of inspiration, replacing my writer's block and fear.

I discovered Ralph Waldo Emerson's poem on the meaning of living a life of success in the Danville Public Library when I was in the fifth or sixth grade. I owe my parents, Dr. Muhammad and Iffat Mushtaq, for instilling a love of books, reading, and education in me, as well as a strong work ethic, from the day I was born. When you are the daughter of immigrants, you see people's unique struggles and sacrifices in creating a life for their families. I grapple with the right words to express my profound gratitude to my parents. As your adult daughter, I desire to honor you and respect the Mushtaq family name by carrying on your compassion, grace, and humility with everyone I serve today. For my brothers and cousins—your messages of support and sharing of comfort food, as I led a nontraditional Desi life, have been a source of laughter and love.

My second family in Danville, the Cunninghams, gave me the nickname Romie. Nate and Theresa Cunningham believed in their daughter, Yanette, and me, in our ability to succeed in school and our lives. During our teenage and adult years, you listened to our personal dramas, and fed us an endless supply of Sara Lee cheesecake and homemade pound cake to share the love. To my childhood bestie, Yanette (Yaddy): Sis, thank you for being one of a handful of people who didn't let me give up when I started my entrepreneurial journey.

Our chosen family, our soul-friends, are the blessings in our lives from Heaven who stay the course of love, and support us through all the changes and stages of our lives. In addition to Yaddy, thank you, Aamira A., Ayesha Z., Brian L., Melissa D., Karen C., Karla F., and my sister-friends for being by my side for years and decades of shared lives.

I dedicated this book to my teachers, starting with my parents and Aunties. My Aunties are my mothers' friends and colleagues, women in our communities from different religions and racial and ethnic backgrounds. They shared similar traditional family values as my parents, and they all helped to raise the collective children of the community together. I am a proud product of a public education school system in a small Midwestern town, Danville, that I am proud to call my hometown. Thank you to all my teachers at Central Christian Pre-School, Liberty Elementary School, North Ridge Middle School, Danville High School, and the after-school programs of the Danville Family YMCA. In the 1980s, young girls were typically guided into home economics and typing classes, but all my teachers understood the assignment. Dr. Mushtaq's daughter would do well in school—math and science were essential on my path to becoming a doctor.

Many professors, doctors, nurses, and hospital administrators gave their time and wisdom to teach me as a medical school student, an internal medicine intern, a neurology resident, and a neurology fellow. Thank you to those who taught me at Fatima Jinnah Medical College, the Medical University of South Carolina, the University of Pittsburgh Medical Center, and the University of Michigan. My heartfelt gratitude and love go to you, Dr. Braxton B. Wannamaker III, Dr. Paul B. Pritchard III, and your families, who have remained teachers, mentors, friends, and extended family members throughout my career.

Let's be honest—I didn't heal or figure out how to heal alone. The Universe brings all of us healers to be light on our path toward growth and self-improvement. I am on my healing journey with a global family of healers who treat the mind, spirit, and physical body. Thank you to Dr. Carlos Pelligrini and the compassionate University of Washington team in Seattle. Thank you to every integrative medicine doctor and colleague who showed me the importance of healing the whole person. Dr. CB Daniel was the first person to hear me after a decade of begging, "I think something is wrong with my thyroid." Thank you for the care since that time, Dr. Thomas Moraczewski; Dr. Annemieke Austin, MD; and Dr. Bindiya Gandhi, MD. We doctors can be difficult and complex patients. You kept me healthy so that I may heal others.

I would not be "here" today without talking to and learning from mental health professionals, including incredible therapists, since I filed for divorce during my fellowship training in 2003. A special prayer of thanks to Karen H., who has been by my side as my therapist for over a decade. My spiritual, mindfulness, meditation, Ayurveda, Reiki, and yoga teachers in the US and around the globe—shukran and namaste.

Thank you, Oprah Winfrey, for modeling what is possible when you lead from your heart and rejoice in fabulous shoes. When I have the chance to meet you in real life, you'll get a larger-than-life thank-you for being the elder sister I always yearned for in my life. I was in middle school when your show went live from WGN studios in Chicago to a national stage. You opened a door for me to learn about the mysteries of US culture as a child of immigrants, along with spirituality and living an authentic life. You continue to model the power of a woman using her voice for the greater good of society.

In 2013, one didn't leave a career in traditional medicine without being labeled insane. I transitioned to a world of integrative medicine, entrepreneurship with an intention to heal teams and individuals. At that time, new mentors, colleagues, and cheerleaders stepped up to guide me even when the path wasn't clear. You all helped raise my consciousness to serve as a visionary, so thank you, Alan Cohen, Karen Drucker, Laurie Young, Martha Beck, Dr. Lissa Rankin, Dr. Sue Mathison, Anne Sharer, Dr. Christine Saba, Pamela Slim, Natalie Mac-Neil, Rabab Al-Amin, Ashley Koff, Suneera Madhani, Sam Horn, and JJ Virgin. Thank you to the TEDxFargo team for allowing me to share my story when people weren't openly talking about mental health and burnout in the workplace.

I can't move further without thanking every person past, present, and future who has worked in or on my business for the Dr. Romie brand and brainSHIFT Institute. Whether you joined us for a few months or years, you shared your heart with the mission. The experience we create for our clients could not have happened without you, Kylie, Cindy, Kyrsten, Mandy, Maggie, and Christian.

Today I have the profound honor to be a part of carrying on Murph's legacy and serve as Evo's Chief Wellness Officer. My favorite Evo guiding principle is "Do everything with gratitude and humility." There are not enough words to express my thank-you for the support and time from the entire senior Evo leadership team, who trusted me to do research, build a company-wide mindfulness program together, and test brainSHIFT. Thank you Murph, Bulmaro, Will, Mary Catherine, Mark, Scott, Brian, Ed, Kris, Gary, Michelle, Matt, and the rest of our corporate leaders. To the thousands of our Evolutionaries who have trusted me with your stories, hopes, and teams—I honor you. I am a better doctor, leader, and human because you welcomed me into your hotels and lives.

Here is a secret about me: I've known since I was in the fourth grade and won the Young Author's Award that I had a book in me. I was *that* girl who dreamed of a book launch party more than a wedding—your actual random and embarrassing fact about me as a gift for reading this far. Publishing houses and agents started reaching out after my TEDxFargo talk got attention, but it never seemed like the right time or fit. And then Peter Joseph, the Editorial Director at Hanover Square Press, contacted me during the global pandemic. Call it my auntie intuition, but even over a Microsoft Teams meeting, I knew his team (and the parent team at HarperCollins) would be the guides to launch *The Busy Brain Cure*. They patiently waited for me to finish the research, test the protocol, and write my first draft of the book. When I randomly emailed Peter at the end of 2021 and said, "I am ready. Let's rock 'n' roll and launch the movement yesterday," he and the team at HarperCollins supported me as a first-time author during the entire process.

Back in early 2013, when I was in a time of paralyzing fear and a Busy Brain over my career transition, Melanie Bates picked up my phone call at a center for integrative medicine training. Melanie was among the first people with whom I shared my painful secret of leaving my career as a traditional neurologist. Even back then, she told me that she couldn't wait to see how my story unfolded. Now she is an absolute badass developmental editor and auntie to stray animals (and authors struggling with writer's block). Your process helped me to unlock my story and share the stories of others, so that everyone reading (and listening) to this book can feel seen and heard while healing their Busy Brains. Every Friday afternoon, your wisdom and laughter helped me to edit my writing and magically gifted Rahja more doggy comfort food. This book was born because of your consummate professionalism and editorial skills—thank you for being my book shaman.

To my beloved dog, Rahja, at sixteen years old. He kept me company for the odd hours I was awake with my Busy Brain to write this book. I know your time is limited on Mother Earth—thank you for making sure I took brain-BREAKs outside to walk with you, got an occasional outing to Starbucks for both of us, and for your snuggles and kisses. Rahja and I hope that you, our readers, know the unconditional love of a soul-dog at least once in your life. In Rahja's honor, a part of the proceeds of this book will be donated to Vanderpump Dogs.

When you assess statistics of who succeeds professionally in the US, the answer differs from someone who looks and thinks like me. I am a daughter of immigrants, learned English as a second language (yes, Dad, technically third), am a recovering burned-out doctor, Desi, and a divorced woman. Yet here I am with a platform to be of service, so I understand the gift God gave me, and I want to give back. It wasn't meant for me to birth human children of my own in this lifetime. Therefore, I want to ensure someone else's daughters are offered every opportunity to be supported. A part of the proceeds of the sale of this book will be donated to the Girl Scouts of Citrus Council in Florida and to the Girl Scouts of the USA. The world of science, technology, engineering, math, and medicine has always lacked diverse voices, and the global pandemic further robbed the pipeline of women and girls. From kindergarten to college to the C-suite, females still lack opportunities for education, mentorship, and leadership. The Girl Scouts is an organization supporting the next generation of glass-ceiling crushers.

And to you, my fellow unapologetic type A, success-driven professionals in our global brainSHIFT community, thank you for trusting me with your brains, hearts, and hopes.